What people are saying about …

THE WISDOM OF YOUR HEART

"Emotions can often be a fickle dish. Still, emotions are made by the finger of God. We are made in the image of God, and as such, we find ourselves in worship before an emotional God who loves, fights, cries, gets jealous, and embodies compassion at every turn of Scripture. Emotions are as central to the life of God as they are to the life of faith. The journey Schelske has trekked here takes us deep into the caverns of these emotions with a fire and fearlessness that I rarely see among Christ followers. I endorse this book heartily. I don't believe it will disappoint."

A. J. Swoboda, PhD, pastor of Theophilus
Church, author of *The Dusty Ones*, and professor
at Portland Seminary and Fuller Seminary

"I'm so grateful there are people like Marc Schelske in the body of Christ who point us to authentic relationships with ourselves and Jesus. *The Wisdom of Your Heart* is a much-needed narrative about the richness we can have in our emotional lives and is full of honest examples and biblical truth."

Mary DeMuth, author of *Worth Living*

"We all need help at times understanding who we are and why we're here. Not long ago, I experienced such a personal crisis, and I wish I would have had this book to guide me."

Jeff Goins, bestselling author of *The Art of Work*

"Despite what you've heard or believed, emotions aren't mere inconveniences that can be buried or brushed aside. Like the determined fly buzzing in your bedroom at night, emotions can be ignored only at the high cost of your rest and peace. Instead, you must acknowledge, listen to, and learn from your emotions. Only then can you find the life of peace and wholeness you crave. This book is the net to help you catch what's been keeping you awake, and Marc is the mentor to help you navigate the dark."

Michele Cushatt, author of *I Am*

"By and large, Western Christianity has exalted the intellect in spiritual matters to the neglect of the emotions. In reaction to this tendency, some Christians have allowed emotions to drive the cart. In *The Wisdom of Your Heart*, Marc Schelske cuts through the fog generated by these two extremes, seeking to set the role of our emotions back in their God-ordained place."

Frank Viola, coauthor of *Jesus Manifesto* and author of *God's Favorite Place on Earth*

THE WISDOM
OF YOUR HEART

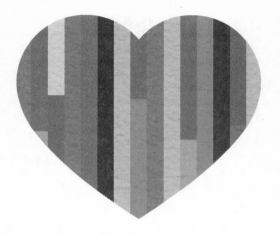

THE WISDOM
OF YOUR HEART

Discovering the God-Given Purpose
and Power of Your Emotions

Marc Alan Schelske

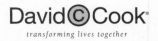
transforming lives together

THE WISDOM OF YOUR HEART
Published by David C Cook
4050 Lee Vance Drive
Colorado Springs, CO 80918 U.S.A.

David C Cook U.K., Kingsway Communications
Eastbourne, East Sussex BN23 6NT, England

The graphic circle C logo is a registered trademark of David C Cook.

The website addresses recommended throughout this book are offered as a resource to you. These websites are not intended in any way to be or imply an endorsement on the part of David C Cook, nor do we vouch for their content.

Details in some stories have been changed to protect the identities of the persons involved.

LCCN 2017933744
ISBN 978-0-7814-1451-7
eISBN 978-0-7814-1465-4

Published in association with literary agent Tawny Johnson of D.C. Jacobson & Associates LLC, an Author Management Company. www.dcjacobson.com.

The Team: Tim Peterson, Keith Wall, Amy Konyndyk, Nick Lee, Jennifer Lonas, Abby DeBenedittis, Julie Neddo, Susan Murdock
Cover Design: Jon Middel
Cover Photo: Getty Images

Printed in the United States of America
First Edition 2017

1 2 3 4 5 6 7 8 9 10

062817

To Christina.
You more than anyone know the words in this book
are the fruit of a long and painful experience. When
I was weak, you carried me in ways that cost you
dearly. It's profoundly insufficient to say I love you.

CONTENTS

PART FOUR: HOW TO HEAR GOD IN YOUR EMOTIONS

PREFACE

Here you are, holding this book, about to decide whether it's right for you. I understand. Reading is a costly investment when our time is overobligated. Before you go any further, I want to tell you where I'm coming from and who might find this book useful.

As these words are published, I am forty-six years old and deep into the most daunting transition of my life. I came to the end of my rope. The tools I built my life with no longer worked. I had been living disconnected from my emotions. Disconnected and afraid. Untended pain leaked out in my relationships. At times I'd see the edges of this darkness and be mortified. I'd want to change—at least I would as long as the pain lasted. I'd read, make lists, rework my schedule, and try some new strategy that promised life change. Invariably some emergency would distract me. How many times can you promise before you're just telling lies? Discouraged, I started believing real change was out of my reach.

Pain forced me to face what I wasn't willing to look at on my own. God was in that pain. I was jarred awake. I knew something had to change—now. I had to do life differently, for my marriage, for my children, and for the church I serve, but most of all for my own emotional and spiritual health.

I'm now several years on from that moment, yet my life still feels caught in the rolling wave of change. I'd like to tell you I've discovered some secret with seven easy steps, but I can't. I can see a better place from here. Some days I even experience a better way of living. This book grew out of everything I've learned in the changing.

I grew up in a conservative Christian home and faith community. Much of that upbringing was good and safe. There I met wise, loving people who shaped me for the better. But as I've entered the second half of life, I'm also learning my background came with baggage: painful experiences, assumptions that have proved untrue, misconceptions about God, even precious habits that turned out to be anything but life giving. I've had to let go of much I used to hold dear. I've also had to learn to grieve those losses.

Years ago I read a book by Pete Scazzero.[1] One line offended me. His words stuck in the back of my mind, like an irritating thorn, forcing me to question myself. "It is not possible," he wrote, "to be spiritually mature while remaining emotionally immature."[2] Could that be true? In four decades, I had never heard this—not in thousands of sermons and youth-group gatherings, in years of Christian education, or in the many leadership conferences I attended. I know I'm not the only one.

Six years ago, I set out to learn everything I could about the emotional life and its connection to spiritual growth. I've traveled through academic writings on the subject of emotions, the body, the brain, and psychology; commentary from generations of theologians and Christian thinkers; and everything I could find in the Bible on the subject. But this journey was intensely personal and practical. I needed to understand my own heart and what God seemed to be doing in my story.

I'm not an expert. I am neither scientist nor therapist. I dug into this subject because I was desperate. I discovered that my own spiritual growth requires facing my emotional brokenness. My journey of maturing in Christ (as we call personal, spiritual, and even emotional growth in the church) has taken me beyond the familiar menu of discipleship made up of Bible study, prayer, service, and worship. These matter, but in my case something was undermining their power—my emotional immaturity. I didn't understand what had happened in my inner world or how that shaped my emotional responses. Like a child, I was expecting other people and outward circumstances to manage my feelings for me. I didn't know how to listen to my emotions. All of this meant I missed growth and wisdom God had for me. As a pastor, I've seen firsthand how the lack of care for emotional wellness hamstrings spiritual growth.

Through this painful process, I've experienced a revitalization of my spiritual life, a kind of conversion leading to a deepening sense of relationship with God. I hope my journey can prove helpful to you. I hope in these pages I can be a trail guide on a tangled path that needs clearing. Perhaps we can cut away some of the obstacles obscuring the path in your own pursuit of wholeness and an intimate relationship with God.

If you feel something missing in your heart, if your relationships continue to struggle no matter how often you promise to be different, if you wrestle with anger, fear, grief, insecurity, or anxiety and wonder whether there is a better way to live, then I invite you to join me on this journey of discovering the wisdom God's placed in your heart.

Marc Alan Schelske

ACKNOWLEDGMENTS

I imagined writers worked in isolation—the ideal craft for an introvert. I was wrong. Good writing is collaborative, a messy potluck assembled by mentors, partners, challengers, colaborers, even innocent bystanders with no idea of the contribution they were making. So here I offer my gratitude to those who made this book possible— at least everyone I can remember today.

Christina, your support of my writing is one of the most concrete expressions of love I've ever experienced. Bridge City, you have been so gracious and generous to me through a long process of evolution. Thank you for cheering me on. Mom, thanks for the love of reading. Byron, your gentle kindness and humble wisdom have been transformative for me. Shelley, you've given me a wonderful model for how to know a lot of things without being a know-it-all. Cindy, as my therapist, you've been a vital link in the possibility of health and hope for me.

Jacqui, your persistent friendship, even though we don't see each other often, gave me great hope when I felt unworthy. Kevin, I don't think anyone has stretched me more toward growth over such a long time. Steven, you caught my hand the moment I was falling off a cliff. Jerry and Ketty, crucial puzzle pieces fell into place at the retreat in your home in Maple Grove. I'm sure you had little idea of the work God was doing in my heart there.

Thanks to other writers who have taken me in and encouraged me. Mary DeMuth, thanks for being an encourager and modeling honest vulnerability. Jeff Goins, thanks for challenging me to get moving. This book wouldn't exist without *You Are a Writer* and the Tribe Writers course. Michele Cushatt, thanks for listening to me in a very raw moment in Vail. Tony Kriz, thanks for pushing the edges of my thinking and becoming a friend. Cornelia Seigneur, thanks for being such a cheerleader, making sure I met all the right people. You are a godsend for an introvert who doesn't enjoy hunting for those people. Brooke Perry, thanks for getting me to my first writers' conference. There would have been no pitch without you.

Thanks to Tawny Johnson, who saw something intriguing in my panicked book pitch, and all the folks at D. C. Jacobson who shepherded these ideas so publishers could catch the vision. Thanks to Tim Peterson and the great team at David C Cook for going to the mat for this book and giving such insightful guidance on how it should be structured.

Oh, and to my beta readers (Michael, Lisa, Christina, Jerry, Cornelia, Byron, Shelley, Cindy), thanks for pushing, asking hard questions, making me clarify, and telling me which stories just didn't land. It was scary inviting you to read the book, but your time and honesty were gifts to me.

It's odd looking at this stack of papers, knowing that while I thought these thoughts and typed these words, none of this would have happened without all of you. For someone who has felt on the outside his whole life, it has given me a sense of place and belonging I've rarely felt before. I had no idea my entourage would be this crowded.

God who creates, Son who walks with us, Holy Spirit who inspires, thank You for all these people.

Thank you all. More than words can say.

Part One

BROUGHT TO A STANDSTILL

Chapter 1

YOU CAN'T RUN FOREVER

We could know, and should know, but don't know because it makes us feel better not to know.

Margaret Heffernan, *Willful Blindness*

My people are destroyed for lack of knowledge.

Hosea 4:6

My chest felt tight. My stomach twisted. Heat rose in my face. I hardened myself against the tears I could tell were coming. I gripped the steering wheel of my car like it was a life preserver. Minutes before, I had been at a breakfast meeting with two church board members. Expectations were crushing me, both my own and those I felt from the church I had pastored for more than a decade. Overwhelmed and overcommitted, I felt like a failure every single day.

If I was going to continue at my church, or in ministry at all, something had to change. How I was working, how I was relating, how I was living—it all needed to change. I needed help, an intimidating admission. I didn't yet realize it, but my sense of value and security was tied to my performance. I couldn't imagine a conversation more painful than telling board members—my bosses—I was failing.

My situation was dire. Anxiously I had asked to meet with these two board members. To prepare, I tracked my working hours in detail for two months—every meeting, task, and project. Surely when they saw this evidence of my overwork, they would help me find a solution.

I shared. They listened. These two men affirmed their support and love for me, but truth be told, they didn't see my crisis. I was just struggling with priorities like anyone in a high-pressure career.

"We all have days we hate our jobs," one said.

They suggested I tweak my hours here or there. One of them told me I ought to spend less time in meetings—while we were in a meeting.

I think these men felt they had helped, but I left the meeting crushed. I felt unheard, even judged as inadequate, hopeless. They didn't intend this; I know they wanted to help. It's often the case, especially when we're wounded, that we hear others inaccurately or interpret their motives unfairly. All I could hear was that I wasn't performing well enough.

I had one tried-and-tested coping mechanism that immediately kicked in: "I'll just work harder to solve this." I started reviewing the tasks I could power through, the hours I could maximize, the steps I could take to change things. But there was no more fuel in the tank. That's when I found myself in my car, unable to hold back the surging waves of tears.

WHERE IS ALL THIS COMING FROM?

Feeling like a failure is painful. Asking for help and not finding it is heartbreaking. But there was another reason this moment was so unsettling. Sitting in a car weeping just wasn't something I did. Ever. A college friend once called me an alien and a pod person because of how little emotion I expressed. I could handle other people's high-pressure crises with levelheaded calm. I was able to reason through a problem without the distraction of emotion.

White-knuckling the steering wheel, I felt out of control. Where was this messy, anxious, angry turmoil coming from? I wasn't used to being overwhelmed like this. In fact, I wasn't used to feeling much at all. No one could see me, yet I felt I was standing naked on a stage, ashamed of my tears.

Judgments swirled in my mind. I was weak for letting this undo me. I just needed to get myself together. I was a bad leader. I should never have talked to the board members; now they would lose confidence in me. I was a poor Christian, with more doubt and fear than faith. I was a fraud. People came to me for counsel, but there I was, a weak and terrified mess.

Few would have predicted I'd be the one to end up weeping in a car. In 1997, I hit the ground running as a staff member for a new church plant. Just two years out of college, I was bursting with ideas, self-confidence, and the unassailable belief I knew what I was talking about. The next ten years were a blaze of productivity and progress. I served in nearly every pastoral role in the church, and I earned accolades as a public speaker. My ministries were growing. At a critical juncture (probably too early), I was asked to serve as senior pastor.

In short order we completed a fund-raiser and bought a building. Everything looked perfect—a young pastor, with a beautiful family, leading a supportive, innovative church.

Behind this image, I'd been living my life at a redline pace. I was involved intimately in nearly every facet of the church's operations. I was available for early-morning breakfast appointments, weekly meetings, counseling sessions at the end of the day, and late-night phone calls to help manage other people's personal crises—which seemed to come up with surprising regularity.

Once or twice a year, though, my wife and I would have a painful conversation about my priorities. Christina felt abandoned. I felt I was just doing my job. She felt I gave my best time to other people. I felt I was serving a higher purpose. How unfair of her to challenge my calling! Her expectations seemed unreasonable to me; my priorities seemed unreasonable to her. She would cry. I'd finally concede. Some current project was demanding too much. As soon as this *one thing* was resolved, life would be different, I'd promise.

When it was just the two of us, I was able to believe my own bright justifications. When our first child, Emerson, was born in 2006, my illusion started to show hairline cracks. Partly, it was the stress all first-time parents experience. No matter how prepared you think you are, you're not. You don't have the emotional resources needed. The never-ending sleep deprivation can push thoughtful, mature adults into something close to mental illness.

But I wasn't willing to admit anything was wrong. Emotions serve in some ways like the warning lights on the dashboards of our cars. Those lights were brightly lit, but I had years of practice ignoring them. Emotion was an unhelpful distraction to bury or set aside, an unbecoming weakness. It would take a divine two-by-four to the head to get my attention.

WHY ARE WE SO DISCONNECTED?

I'm not the only one. People all around us are going through the motions of life emotionally disconnected. Some live with an encasing numbness, feeling little at all. Others are numb only to the highs of joy and the depths of sorrow. This was my experience for years. Living without emotion, or with suppressed emotion, is terrible and terribly common. In fact, 16.1 million Americans reported having an episode of depression in 2015,[1] but there are many more who wouldn't use that word to describe their experience. We look productive, but our interior lives are stretched thin. We experience only a narrow range of semifeelings, leaving us emotionally hobbled.

Think of the single mom who sprints through her overobligated daily life, ignoring pervasive sadness. Consider the hard-driving CEO who disconnected from his feelings years ago, because "you can never let them see you sweat." Then there's the even-keeled church volunteer masking icy anger behind his polite silence.

How did this come about? We've experienced a long, consistent attack on our emotional selves. We don't even realize how we've come to look down on this critical part of our lives.

Try a little experiment with me, will you? I'm going to ask you to say a simple sentence aloud. Say it as you might in a conversation. When you do, notice how it feels. Ready? Here's the sentence:

You seem really reasonable today.

How do those words feel? Imagine how they would feel if you were saying them to someone else. Imagine someone else saying these words to you. Hold on to the feeling for a moment.

Now I have a second sentence for you. Try this one out and see how it feels:

You seem really emotional today.

How did this second sentence feel? How would it feel if someone said these words to you? Now compare the two sentences. They feel different, don't they?

When I've done this exercise with groups of people, they invariably give the same response. Being called reasonable feels like a compliment. Being called emotional feels like criticism. In just ten words, we've unearthed something true about our culture.[2] Many of us hold a belief we may not even be aware of. It goes like this:

> *Reason* is good, a quality to be admired and sought after. Someone who is reasonable is among the grown-ups who can be trusted with important things. *Emotion* is bad, or at least untrustworthy. An emotional person is flighty or immature, someone who can't be trusted to think clearly when it matters.

These voices are in your head. They're certainly in mine. "You can't trust your emotions. You don't want to make an emotional decision. Just be reasonable."

The culture we've grown up in has made a god of reason. This worship has deep roots, reinforced over and over throughout history. Plato taught that emotion and reason are always at war. He likened emotion to an untamed horse. Reason provided the reins for keeping emotions in check.[3]

The Stoic philosophers, like Seneca, taught that emotions are the result of thinking errors. They encouraged the pursuit of *apatheia*, a state of no passion.[4] If that sounds vaguely familiar, it should. It's the root of the English word *apathy*, not caring at all.

René Descartes, the father of modern philosophy, famously said, "I think; therefore I am." This single sentence reduces the measure of our existence to rational thought.

Some scientists have wondered whether emotions are the residual effect of evolutionary history. These instincts kept us alive when predators chased us across the African plains, but perhaps they're becoming obsolete.

Many religious communities see discipline, self-control, and doing the right thing as markers of spiritual maturity.

We've taken these lessons to heart, accepting emotions as second-class citizens in the mature and responsible soul. As if that isn't enough, painful life circumstances taught many of us that powerful emotions are trouble. Perhaps like me, you've experienced profound loss or trauma that disrupted your childhood. Maybe you were abused or experienced enormous loss in some other way. A friend of mine who experienced shocking abuse as a child once told me the implicit motto of his life had become "Don't talk. Don't trust. Don't feel."

We've learned from our culture, from our institutions, and from our own painful experiences that emotions just aren't safe. Matthew Elliott, in his book *Feel*, wrote,

> For years we've been taught by our culture and in our churches that emotions are not to be trusted; that reason and knowledge and logic are the firm foundation on which to build our faith and our spiritual lives.[5]

If this is true, then living a spiritual life means practicing self-control, managing our emotions instead of letting them manage us. To be fair, there's something to this idea. We've all made terrible decisions based on how we felt at the time. We've seen loved ones follow their feelings into destructive relationships or terrible habits. Parents fear their children will make important decisions emotionally. Countless bad choices have been justified with a sincere "It just feels right."

With all this harm, it's not a surprise when churches make the connection between emotion and sin. People get emotional and then do something on our sin list. It looks almost like cause and effect. We make a conclusion that seems obvious: Emotions are, at best, a distraction. At worst, they are self-deception, not a gift but a curse. No mature, healthy, or spiritual decision can be made following our emotions.

Pete Scazzero is one of the rare pastors who is known for including emotional health and growth in the normal process of discipleship in the church. In his groundbreaking book *Emotionally Healthy Spirituality*, he shares how, even as a pastor, he had been steeped in this negative perception of emotions. He writes, "Like most Christians, I was taught that almost all feelings are unreliable and not to be trusted. They go up and down and are the last thing we should be attending to in our spiritual lives."[6]

Our goal, which seems so good, so Christian, is to live by what is true, not by what we feel. If we want to be mature and faithful, then we must ignore fickle emotions. Of course the emotions of fallen, sinful creatures are untrustworthy. If emotions can lead us to hurt others, make selfish decisions, or disobey God in a hundred other ways, we need to overcome them, right? The only seemingly righteous path left is ignoring or denying our emotions. I've come across this idea in more books and sermons than I can remember. I believed it for a long time. I've even preached it.

Once, I was counseling a church member going through intense grief. She said with passion, "Wouldn't it just be better if we could turn off our emotions? We could obey God better without all these feelings." Her desire to stop feeling pain was normal, but her conclusion was misguided.

Our lack of emotional maturity does great harm. Consider the pastor who counsels an abused wife to just let her loving attitude change her husband. Or the men's ministry leader who tells the abuser to just "read the Bible and pray more" to control his anger. Or the Christian leader so deep in denial that he finds himself living an unsustainable double life that eventually collapses in a gruesome display of moral failure. Failures like these are the fruit of our inability to talk about, process, and understand our emotions.

This silence keeps couples from knowing each other and contributes to the failure of marriages. It infiltrates our parenting. It has kept good people stuck in eddies of spiritual stagnancy. It shuts up our hearts, locking down our intuition. We become more and more brittle. Something is wrong with this situation!

Here's the truth: God didn't create us as beings of pure reason who happen to be burdened by the glandular effects of irrational emotion. We'll turn to Scripture soon, and there you'll see that God created us as whole beings—body, mind, and spirit. All of that was made in God's image. Let me be clear: this includes your emotions.

In case you've never heard that before, I'll repeat it. Your emotions are made in God's image too.

QUESTIONS FOR REFLECTION

You'll find questions for reflection at the end of every chapter. Take time to think them through. Ideally, you'll journal your reflections and then pray over what you've written. This will help you more deeply engage with the material. You may even hear God speaking as you do.

In addition to these questions, you can find additional material at www.TheWisdomOfYourHeart.com that supports each chapter, recommended reading, downloadable resources, and online small-group and individual courses to help you grow.

1. Were you taught that emotions are unreliable or untrustworthy? Where did this message come from in your life?

2. What feelings surfaced when you spoke the two test sentences aloud: "You seem really reasonable today" and "You seem really emotional today"? Why do you think you had the reaction you did?

3. Think about the woman who asked whether our lives would be better if we could just turn off our emotions. If this were possible, how would your life be different? How might it improve things for you? How would it make things worse? How might this affect your life of faith?

Chapter 2

A CRAZY PROPHET AND MY HIDDEN SHATTERING

The past is never where you think you left it.

Katherine Anne Porter, *Ship of Fools*

God, create a clean heart for me and renew a steadfast spirit within me.

Psalm 51:10

Emotions are made in God's image? I didn't believe this for most of my life. I had emotions—we all do. But I felt uncomfortable with most of mine. I was numb to the rest.

Accomplishment had given me a sense of personal value. I'm a hard worker, responsible, with high personal initiative. As a student, as a volunteer, and then as a pastor, I earned respect and affirmation based on my performance. Whenever life got painful, I would retreat to this well-worn path of discipline and hard work. Find the cause. Solve the problem. The cost didn't matter.

I was thirty-six. I'd served my church as a pastor for ten years by then, three as the senior pastor. I had been married for almost seven years. Life seemed on the right track. The church was bouncing along fine. Fine, but not growing—not in numbers, not in depth either. It seemed to take more and more effort to keep the ball rolling. I had an amazing and supportive staff. We had committed volunteers, yet I couldn't connect deeply with most of them. In the quiet corners of my heart, I knew something was wrong, but I just kept pushing hard down the path I knew. Try harder. Perform better. Get it right.

I hoped these painful questions, like ghostly images fluttering in my peripheral vision, would fade away. Then something happened that shook me deeply. It was something I didn't really even believe in.

"TWO THINGS THE LORD WANTS TO SAY"

I was visiting a friend's church on a quick out-of-town getaway. After the service, a woman wanted to speak with me. My friend warned me. This might be weird, he said. The woman was either mentally ill or a prophet. A prophet. Like in the biblical sense. Not inspirational thoughts, but actual messages from God.

My first inclination was to pass, but what if this was the real deal? Just because I had never experienced a personal prophetic message before didn't mean it was impossible. A tight heaviness developed in my gut. I didn't realize this was anxiety surfacing. I wanted to make it go away, but discomfort seemed a flimsy excuse for not hearing this woman out. If she were crazy, listening to her words couldn't hurt me, right?

As the congregation dispersed, I sat next to her in an empty row of chairs. In the background, the musicians were noisily packing up their gear.

"There are two things the Lord wants to say to you today." That's how she started. No messing around.

"First, within a year you will have a son, and the Lord will use that son to soften your heart and expand your ability to care for people."

At this point, my daughter wasn't even a year old. Life with a newborn had stretched Christina and me beyond our capacity. If we were going to have a son within a year, well, we would need to get that project underway in the next couple of months. Frankly, that was the furthest thing from our minds. I started sliding this woman over into the mentally ill category.

"Second, the Lord says you are the reason your church is not growing," she declared. "If you don't allow God to change your heart, your church will die." Dead stop.

True or not, those were fighting words. Apart from my family, there was nothing I loved more than my church. I'd been with the church through agonizing trauma and exuberant victory. The health of the church was in my thoughts and prayers every single day. With this woman's absurd suggestion that we'd have a son within a year and her offensive accusation, I was done listening to her. I thanked her for her time and excused myself, wondering what my friend had gotten me into.

I didn't think about the crazy prophet woman again until just about a year later. On a bright Sunday morning in October of 2007, Christina and I brought our son, Lucas, home from the hospital. Earlier that summer, we'd begun the complicated process of applying to adopt. We planned for an international adoption. The first step was a home study with a local agency. In the best scenario we could imagine, we might complete the home study, apply for an adoption, and have a baby eighteen months or even two years in the future—if there were no bumps in the road.

But as our home study concluded in July, the local agency called us. It was a small Christian agency and didn't have any families prepared to adopt a little boy due in October. Were we willing to switch from an international adoption to be considered for this local child who needed a family?

It would be an understatement to say everything went smoothly. Lucas was born in October, not even ninety days after that call. We brought him home from the hospital three days later, an almost unheard-of timeline for domestic adoptions. Our heads were spinning. It seemed almost miraculous.

Somewhere in the chaos of those weeks, the words I had heard nearly a year before crashed into my consciousness.

"Within a year you will have a son ..."

What? This couldn't be right. That woman couldn't possibly have been speaking for God. Yet here I was holding a son who hadn't even entered my mind just three months before.

Now arose a painful question. Was this woman right about her second message? Was the first message God's way of validating what would be too painful for me to consider otherwise? Was I really the bottleneck preventing growth in the church I loved? Were my failures so terrible the church would die if I didn't change?

I knew I wasn't a perfect pastor. My shortcomings were many. I found strategies, plans, and tasks easier than relating to people. I was losing myself in administrative projects rather than facing the difficult conversations of pastoral care. I was altogether too confident of my own ideas and too easily overlooked the counsel of others. As an introvert, I required enormous amounts of emotional energy to be on my game every weekend, available for anyone who needed me.

I had been working on these deficits for years, and it seemed I was making headway. People I had worked with or served said they had seen me grow. Were my rough edges so sharp they would do my church in? This question stalked and harried me, a beast of fear and regret, terrifying to confront. I wanted to run, avoid, quickly skirt the issue. I would have if I could have held myself together.

FALLING APART UNSEEN

When Christina and I brought Lucas home, those cracks forming in my life widened dangerously. I was committed to being a good husband—at least in my mind. I was committed to being a good pastor in spite of my fears. I was committed to being a good father. In my sleep-deprived, ragged, overextended state, the pressure of those commitments rolled down on me in crushing waves.

There was no way I could succeed. To keep one commitment in the way I thought I needed to meant I failed at another. I felt blind. I forgot things, missed appointments. The plates I had kept spinning in the air for so long started crashing to the ground. With each failure, my self-esteem fragmented.

I'd sit at my desk, stuck, knowing if I could just finish a task, I'd feel better, but I often couldn't. I'd head home feeling like a failure at work. Then after arriving later than promised, I'd look in Christina's tired eyes and feel like a failure in my marriage.

My internal landscape darkened. At one point, for months and months, I hardly had the courage to get out of bed in the morning. When I did make it to work, unable to focus, I'd spend hours on a project that should have taken twenty minutes. I'd escape through media, busywork, and administrative trivia that made me feel as if I was accomplishing something. For the first time since I was a child, I was losing control of my life. Pain was seeping through my defenses.

I didn't understand what was happening to me. If you had asked what I was feeling, I couldn't have told you. Sometimes I was numb. The only emotion I could identify was anger. Most of the time I didn't dare call it by that name. I'd say I was irritated or frustrated or disappointed. I rarely felt happy or joyful. I felt alone and afraid. I became more insecure and inflexible. I had never been good at intimacy, and fear made me impenetrable.

I was reading the Bible and journaling, praying like mad, begging God for some light. It all felt like meaningless gestures. When I could muscle up motivation, I'd work even harder, but it didn't change anything, and I'd collapse again.

At one point I fell into a sick weekly cycle. I'd work hard and fast, writing my sermon, preparing details for the worship team, and connecting with leaders so groups could run smoothly. When the weekend arrived, I'd get up at three in the morning to finalize my notes and prepare for a seventeen-hour day at church. I'd leave everything out on the stage, giving my best good-pastor performance; then I'd drag myself home and collapse. I wouldn't be able to function in any meaningful way until Tuesday. I'd spend Wednesday in a mental fog, fighting to pull myself back together so the process could begin again for the next weekend. This went on for months.

Because I was such a high performer, because so few people knew the state of my heart, and because I was desperate, clutching the last shreds of personal identity built on accomplishment and strength, it never occurred to me or anyone around me (except perhaps my wife) that I was in the middle of a deep, smothering depression.

I could see what mattered most to me was slipping away. My relationship with Christina was barreling toward a cliff. I treated my children with harsh impatience. I felt emotionally numb, the numbness masking a cauldron of bitter frustration. My spiritual life was dry and difficult. For all of this, I felt enormous shame. I could see where this road was taking me. The consequences were too great. Something had to change.

WE LIVE OUR STORIES, OR OUR STORIES LIVE US

During this time, I became good friends with a man named Byron, who happened to be a trauma therapist. He challenged me with an idea: he told me that we all live our lives out of our stories.

Our stories, in the way he was using the word, are the narratives we hold about our own lives. Our stories are the history of our experiences, but they're more than that. They're the web of meaning, explanation, and even justification that we've woven around our memories and history. Much of the time, without even knowing it, we choose to live out of these stories.

We see this with women who were abused as children—they repeatedly seek out relationships with abusive men. Then there are those young adults raised in fundamentalist religious homes who, despite all their parents' efforts, go off the deep end in self-destructive rebellion. These stories, clichés in how often they occur, are just extreme examples of what is true for all of us.

Sometimes we react to our stories, pushing away from what happened to us. Other times we reenact them, living out what is most familiar, even if it's painful. Sometimes we try to resolve something unresolved within us, searching for the love or affirmation that was missing from our childhoods. In many cases, we express our stories in our attitudes, emotions, and choices. If you don't know and understand your own story, it will keep shaping your choices.

In my pastoral role, I often get to hear people's personal stories. After almost two decades of this, I'm convinced most people don't know why they do what they do. Christian people sometimes think bad things continue to happen in their lives because they don't pray enough or because they aren't trying hard enough. We project these same beliefs onto others, judging their choices as selfish, hypocritical, or simply lazy. Those assessments may be accurate at times, but there's something else to consider. We all do what we do for reasons. Those reasons are rooted in our stories.

Sometimes we aren't aware of this, and all it takes to free us from destructive patterns is understanding. Other times it takes the careful guidance of a therapist or spiritual director to help us face our stories in a process of healing that may take years.

Our stories can obstruct the path to growth, the path to mature relationships. Deeply rooted habits, as well as ongoing brokenness and sin, can keep us from seeing the truth about ourselves. We hear people in church talk about the abundant life, but we don't have a grasp on it ourselves. Maybe we even wonder whether there is such a thing. Perhaps it's just the superspiritualized language of Christians who are good at pretending everything is fine.

I'd seen all of this in the lives of people I worked with and pastored. It's so easy to see in others! But I hadn't given much attention to my own story and how my past had shaped me and my struggle with emotions.

I thought I was mostly fine. I wasn't.

A CLUE IN MY STORY

My story was driving me. In February of 2011, I found myself in a circumstance where I unexpectedly got to see into my own heart. God set it up—there's no question in my mind.

A few months prior, I had begun sharing my struggle with another pastor. Steven had been through some of the most horrible abuse imaginable. That led him to become a superperformer. After one church plant came to a painful end, he was forced to face his own sickness. Because of his experience, he could see right through my denial and justification. He was crass, painfully direct, and a little too willing to get involved in other people's dramas. But he probably saved my life.

Steven didn't judge me, but he wouldn't corroborate my story either. He told me the truth about where I was. He told me I had a life-and-death decision to make. I couldn't fix myself. I had to get help. I was horrified to be seen in this way, but being seen like this *and* being cared for? That felt like hope, like someone having hope for me when I couldn't hold on to hope for myself.

I agreed to go on a small pastoral retreat with Steven and a couple of others. The retreat, led by a therapist and former pastor named Jerry, was for ministry leaders experiencing burnout. It didn't sound like fun at all, but I was willing to try just about anything— even if it required flying to Minnesota in the middle of winter for a touchy-feely retreat.

At one point the facilitator gave us a personality inventory. I love these! Boxing up reality into neatly labeled categories is a hobby of mine. When the results came back, however, I noticed something strange. In this particular inventory, I had scored high as someone who processes life in my head—intellectual, linear, an objective thinker. That rang true. But I also scored high as a person who processed life intuitively, emotionally, in my gut. Someone else might have just blown this off. After all, words on paper don't define us. But I was frustrated because I'd had this experience before. On other personality inventories, I had gotten the same kind of seemingly contradictory result. And each time, the counselor or adviser would just say, "Huh. That's weird. We don't normally see this."

The retreat group was sitting in the living room talking about our inventory results. I was venting. I needed to make sense of this discrepancy. The day before, Jerry the Therapist had talked about emotional learning. He said that personality is in some ways just a collection of deeply ingrained habits. These habits are formed during our preverbal and early childhood as we tackle a number of essential tasks.

We're all looking for love, security, and a sense of belonging. We try different strategies to fill these needs. When something seems to work, we keep doing it. When something doesn't work, especially in a painful or traumatic way, we avoid that path in the future. Even before we know this is happening, we learn strategies for how to be accepted, how to feel valuable, and how to get what we need. We learn these lessons so early, they become nearly hardwired into our systems. They're so habitual, we think of them as part of our personalities. Experiences of intense stress or trauma crystalize this emotional learning even more rapidly. The more viscerally emotional the experience, the deeper the lesson is wired into our psyches.[1]

A visceral experience of trauma? I had one of those. I can still remember the images, words, and feelings as if they happened this week. My dad, the sole pastor of a busy church, never ran out of work to do. One August morning when I was eleven, he left the house early to catch up on his to-do list at the office. It was his day off. I never saw him alive again. A fall from a ladder while cleaning his second-story office window shattered my family, ending my childhood.

I've always known this was one of my deepest formative influences. Sitting frustrated in that living room in Minnesota, I felt there was more in that experience for me to look at, but I had a problem. I couldn't remember many substantive details about myself before the day my dad died. I could remember that historical event in crisp detail, but I didn't have any access to my own sense of what I was like before it happened.

There was one other unique aspect of this pastoral retreat. As I mentioned, Jerry the Therapist was a former pastor, well equipped to speak into the issues this difficult vocation brings with it. I didn't mention that he was also my uncle by marriage. His wife, Ketty, was my mother's youngest sister. She had lived with my family a number of summers before my dad died.

I had forgotten this entirely. She was a teenager then, my favorite aunt.

At that moment, while I was venting to the others at the retreat about not being able to recall what I was like before my dad died, Ketty was cooking dinner for all of us. Here was one of the few people in the world who knew what I needed to know.

My aunt joined our conversation. She told me how she had experienced me as an energetic, joyful kid who was always making things. She remembered me as creative, sensitive, and soft. She teared up as she shared her clear sense that when my dad died, something changed. I shifted, became different—responsible, right, careful, in charge. My heart closed safely behind a door.

Her words felt like God gently speaking to my heart. Puzzle pieces clicked. Here I was, decades later, well practiced at being a "head person," suspicious of emotion, both controlling and controlled. In a crisis I was the person others wanted around. I didn't lose my head. I didn't get emotional. Holding things together while others fell apart became a central facet of my identity, a story I would reenact over and over.

This came at great cost, however. I could keep the train on the tracks, but I couldn't grieve my own losses. I could organize systems and manage projects, but I couldn't connect intimately even with the people I loved most. But here was a clue. Maybe this way of being wasn't my whole identity! As I flew home to Portland, a new sense of possibility opened up for me. I felt enormous hope. Well, in truth, I felt hope and fear. It seemed to me for the first time in a long time that God had showed up in my life.

Maybe my need to keep order, to carefully manage and control my world, to organize away the chaos, wasn't entirely the truth about who I was. Maybe my discomfort with intuition (even my own) and my belief that emotions were untrustworthy were less about my personality and more about trying to avoid pain. If this was true, I needed to understand and experience my emotions in a different way.

It turned out that would be hard to do.

QUESTIONS FOR REFLECTION

1. Because of my backstory, accomplishment and performance became my primary path for building a sense of value and security in my life. For some, the path to value and security is being right. For others, value and security come from being needed. Do you have a sense of what your primary path for creating value and security is? How do you think this came to be in your life?

2. Our stories (the narratives of our lives and the meanings we've given them) shape our lives deeply. Until we're conscious of this, we tend to live either reacting to our stories ("I will never be like my dad!") or reenacting them ("I feel most comfortable around strong women—like my mom"). Sometimes we do both. Do you see one or both of these forces at work in your life today?

3. How might your story have led you into brokenness, unhealthy habits, or even sin? How has it shaped your experience of emotion?

Chapter 3

A KILLER GPS

If the map doesn't agree with the ground, the map is wrong.
Gordon Livingston, *Too Soon Old, Too Late Smart*

Can the blind guide the blind? Won't they both fall into a pit?
Luke 6:39

I had never been to New York City before. Of course Christina and I were thrilled when a conference took us there. We flew in at night. Looking out the window before landing, I could see city lights stretching out forever. This city is in a completely different league!

My first experience of the subway confirmed my suspicion with gritty certainty. We were headed to a Broadway show, so we took the subway at a corner station near our hotel. But we had to make a transfer at Grand Central Station.

Our train hurtled into the underground station, creaking as it stopped. As I stepped out of the train, my brain went into sensory overload. The echoing clatter and screech of trains along with the urgent press of people assaulted us. Three other tracks ran beside ours, but the train we needed wasn't on any of them. We rushed down an ancient flight of stairs. More tracks and more trains, but our train wasn't there either. We took another flight of stairs even deeper. Finally, four levels beneath the street, we found our train. Grand Central is like an enormous heart pumping the flow of people through the city. So many trains, so many tracks, so many levels. I couldn't make any sense of it.

Fortunately, we live in the age of smartphones with geolocation. In short order, Christina had downloaded an app to guide us through the tangle. We needed that map to make sense of where we were. GPS devices and mapping apps on our smartphones have made it easy to navigate unfamiliar territory. Until they don't work right.

For years, Google's data was used in the dominant mapping apps, but in 2012, Apple stopped using Google's data in its new Apple Maps. The app was beautifully designed, but it had one small problem. The mapping data the app initially depended on was flawed.[1] Streets were missing. Location data was attached to the wrong addresses. Stories of mapping failures poured in from frustrated users. For more than a year, skiers headed to the Pennsylvania mountains kept showing up in Judy Saltsburg's driveway, thinking they were on the best route to a nearby ski lodge.[2] Travelers trying to get to Alaska's Fairbanks International Airport were routed onto the runway.[3] Police in Victoria, Australia, warned tourists to stop using Apple Maps after several were stranded in the Outback for twenty-four hours without enough food or water.[4]

These misguided folks weren't to blame for ending up in the wrong places. They were traveling in unfamiliar territory. They needed a map to find their way, but the map they were given was flawed. Flawed maps are untrustworthy. They can even be dangerous.

THE EMOTIONAL MAPS WE INHERIT

In life we get handed maps. These maps aren't often on paper or on our mobile devices, yet we rely on them when we find ourselves in unfamiliar territory. We collect relational maps, family maps, cultural maps. Most we inherit during childhood from people we love and trust, people who seem to know what they're talking about. In this way, parents, teachers, pastors, and mentors begin to shape the future course of our lives.

Sometimes these maps are helpful; sometimes they are useless. Here's one example. My father was a well-respected leader, conscientious and hard working. Watching him gave me a map of what responsible manhood looked like. However, my father died when I was eleven. He never taught me how to shave or talked with me about relationships. In these unfamiliar places, the map I inherited was just a bare sketch.

The map of manhood I got from my father was flawed in other ways too. He grew up in a traditional farming family on the North Dakota plains, with an unexpressive German father. Affection wasn't part of their relationship. My dad never heard his father tell him he loved him or even that he was proud of him. Dad was affectionate with us, however. Somehow he had decided to change this pattern from his childhood. But in other ways, his emotions were tightly managed. He would never lash out in anger, retreating instead behind a wall of icy silence. Sometimes he was passive-aggressive. This map I received from my father wasn't able to guide me toward emotional maturity.

FOUR WAYS THE CHRISTIAN MAP OF EMOTIONS IS OFTEN WRONG

Many of the mental maps I inherited came from the church community I grew up in. I had an implicit set of beliefs about the role of emotions in the life of a Christian. These weren't always explicit lessons taught in classrooms or sermons. My maps were a jumble of intuitions, preconceptions, prejudices, and beliefs I gleaned from family, teachers, and youth pastors. They were drawn from passing warnings, judgmental glances, and whispered gossip about kids who were heading down the wrong track.

Not every church community is like this. Some faith communities and denominational traditions are much more affirming of emotions. Many people grew up without this baggage. Yet I've talked about this topic with so many others who grew up in church, and I learned that these beliefs weren't unique to me. This shared cultural map comprises four different but connected myths.

These myths often go unquestioned. Having learned them in church, we assume they're biblical. They aren't. Yet they carry such authority, many of the people who shared their stories with me felt as if they were poor Christians or even sinful when their lives didn't measure up. Like any flawed map, these flawed beliefs mislead. Not only are they wrong; they're also destructive.

1. Emotions Always Lie

"Whatever you do, don't make an emotional decision!" With this admonition, youth pastors and teachers in the church I grew up in tried to steer us kids away from bad choices and bad behavior. "If you're on a date and the evening's winding down, everything will feel good," they told us. "Sitting in the back seat of the car together will seem like the best possible thing to do. But you can't make a decision then. Your emotions will lead you astray. You'll be pulled right into sin! You may wind up with an STD or pregnant. You'll undermine your witness. The only way you can make good decisions is to make them when you're clearheaded and unemotional."

How many times have you heard advice like this? It's wise. We can all name people who followed their emotions right off a cliff. Emotions spike with intensity. They move us, and then we act, often in shortsighted, even self-destructive ways. Parents, pastors, and teachers only wanted to keep us from making life-altering, bad decisions. Their protective advice was just common sense, right?

The problem, we were told, is that our emotions always lie to us. Despite all our training and good intentions, emotions can lead us to feel certain choices are right, even godly. The feeling will be powerful. It will feel real, but it will be deceptive. This message was so deeply embraced that the very idea of following our feelings was practically synonymous with doing something sinful.

Jeremiah 17:9 (NIV) was quoted often: "The heart is deceitful above all things and beyond cure. Who can understand it?" The clear message I heard in church was that emotions would blind us to what was true and lead us into danger. There was no wisdom to be found there. As kids, we were warned to avoid the catastrophe of Romans 1, where certain horrible sinners had "exchanged the truth of God for a lie."[5] Undoubtedly our emotions would lead us down this road. We were to be people of truth. This meant being careful not to let emotions influence us.

As with all myths, this one has a core of truth. Emotions do influence us deeply, and sometimes that influence seems against our best interests, perhaps even against God's will. We can easily misunderstand and misattribute emotions. We can overreact or ignore them. We can do all of this because we're immature emotionally and, of course, because we're sinful. This is the true message of Jeremiah 17:9—not that emotions are entirely untrustworthy but that we are sinful and full of unending reasons to justify our behavior.[6] As such, we can follow feelings blindly into trouble and then blame them when the consequences come our way. But as we'll see in the coming chapters, our core emotional responses are not lies. They are almost always telling us something true and important about our inner landscapes or outer circumstances.

2. Emotions Are Always Shallow and Transitory

Another reason we were taught to avoid making emotional decisions was because of how quickly emotions changed. If you experienced a feeling that was uncomfortable—or worse, seemed out of line with God's will—you were to double down on what you knew to be true. Ignore the emotion, and it would go away. That was often called living by faith. We were taught to keep the proper sequence: faith, fact, feelings, in that order. There was no encouragement to stop and reflect on the feelings we were having. Why would you? You were going to feel differently tomorrow.

Now, there are certainly times in the life of faith when we lean into what we believe about God. There are moments when the right road is the hard road, when conviction carries us through uncertainty. And yet, in suggesting that emotions were never more than a passing urge or impulse, we forced faith to take on a hard-edged, linear rationality.

My church measured faith in intellectual terms. Our precious spiritual practices were memorizing Scripture, debating theology, and defending our faith through apologetics. The more a preacher used Greek and Hebrew and taught the meat of systematic theology, the better he (always he) was. Even our music was intellectual. Either it was the old hymns, with six verses of dense theology, or classical music, which was superior because, like math or literature (I was told), it edified the mind.

We looked down on our charismatic brethren. With their rock-'n'-roll music and loud, emotional outpourings, they were at best immature. At worst, they were misled. Their shallow worship services didn't have the meat and grandeur ours did. Our public prayers were carefully thought through, articulate, and theologically accurate rather than spontaneous, heartrending, and *embarrassing*. Except maybe in the youth group or the women's ministry meeting, where a certain amount of emotionalism was expected and, well, unavoidable, right?

This is a bit of an exaggeration, but not much. Our need to avoid shallow emotion required us to redefine some important biblical concepts—and take the feelings out. Joy, for example, was explained as an experience more profound than happiness. Happiness was shallow, rooted in circumstances; it would come and go. Joy, on the other hand, was something a follower of Jesus could choose, a state of mind any good Christian could live in, regardless of their feelings. We could have joy even when we felt sad or unhappy! *Agape* love was also not a shallow or passing feeling. This kind of love was a willful choice we made to follow Jesus' example of self-sacrifice. This was more dependable than the inconsistent, often volatile emotion of love.

These transitory emotions were just not trustworthy. We needed something solid. In the church of my childhood, that meant relying instead on established doctrinal interpretations. It meant staying faithful to our community's moral standards. It meant doing what was right because it was right. In fact, that was the highest definition of a godly person: someone who would go against culture, who would face down opposition, who would even *go against his or her own feelings* to do what was right.

Even now, those words sound so righteous—to follow God's will in spite of your own feelings. But what about the times your understanding of God's will is wrong? What about the times the Holy Spirit moves you to do something hard or unexpected, something that challenges a teaching you thought you understood? In the coming chapters, we'll discover that our emotions always bring messages from our deepest inner places and that with a mature understanding tempered by scriptural wisdom, they are not to be lightly disregarded.

3. God Isn't Emotional

I remember seeing a Jesus movie as a kid. In this film, Jesus was haunting, dour, and always calm. His long blond hair hung loose around His gaunt face, framing blue eyes. He spoke quietly. His words formed succinct, wise sentences as if He knew they would eventually be recorded in Scripture. To my young eyes, He seemed distant and unmoved.

If Jesus was aloof, though, that was an improvement over His Father. At least Jesus had a tangible body and made the effort to walk around in sandals. In my imagination, God was a much-larger-than-scale, ancient patriarch with a giant white beard. He was robed in power and majesty, whatever that meant. He was the creator who sustained the universe. With a mind more powerful than all the computers and all the networks in the world, He was able to hear every prayer, consider every sparrow, and keep all the galaxies spinning safely. This God was completely *other*, completely *beyond*.

Emotions? God had nothing whatsoever to do with them. I don't think anyone ever said this exactly, but that's the picture I got. I was taught that God is holy and just. The Bible awkwardly mentioned that God gets angry, even jealous. But that didn't mean God was emotional!

I learned that our emotions—love, fear, anger, joy—are all fickle, and God is not fickle. God is unchanging.[7] Emotions can derail us from our good intentions and lead us into temptation, but "God is not tempted by evil."[8] This meant, at least in my mind, that God doesn't really have emotions.

Those who taught me the Bible affirmed this. The emotional language in Scripture, they said, wasn't a matter of feelings. These were statements about God's character. For example, God's kind of love—*agape*—described God's act of sacrifice. God's anger also had a special name—*wrath*—which was God's ultimate justice. These words weren't emotions. They described God's unchanging character and the actions God would take. God was "the unmoved mover," beyond having passions like these.

This perspective made God safe. A God untouched by emotion seemed trustworthy. We didn't have to worry about unexpected rage or jealousy. If we needed God to have feelings, we could separate out those duties and give them to Jesus. He was human, after all. Jesus could have some feelings, certainly the holy ones. But God the Father? No. God was unmovable.

As safe as this view of God seemed, it turns out to be the furthest thing from Scripture. Later in this book, we'll look closely at what the Bible says and reveal the truth about this myth.

4. The More Godly You Become, the Less Emotional You'll Be

Like a simple math problem, these first three myths added up to one obvious conclusion: the more like God you become, the less emotional you will be.

Christians strive to be more godly. Ephesians 4:11–13 tells us that God is working to grow us up in the image of Christ. We'd sing, "Be like Jesus, this my song, in the home and in the throng; be like Jesus, all day long! I would be like Jesus."[9] The youth version was simpler but carried the same message: "I want to be more like You. I want to be a vessel You work through. I want to be more like You."[10]

Jesus wasn't just our savior. He was our model. Being like Jesus was our goal. While we were all sinners, prone to constant failure, we also knew we should emulate Jesus. This was always the right choice. After all, WWJD?

God was truth and spoke only truth. God was solid and dependable. We thought God was everything our emotions were not. If God wasn't emotional, didn't that mean our emotions weren't spiritual either?

Maybe emotions were sinful, something to resist. Or maybe they were an unfortunate reality of life in these bodies, something that would disappear when we're made new. In the meantime, emotions were something to manage. They weren't a part of our spiritual lives. At least that's what I thought.

Again, no one at church ever said this out loud, but it got telegraphed all the time. People who expressed extreme grief embarrassed us, especially if their grief lasted too long. People who were too happy creeped us out a little. As I shared before, my tribe of believers didn't trust the charismatic Christians who were always talking about how God made them feel. More than one pastor I knew made fun of those "Jesus is my girlfriend" praise choruses, which they claimed lacked any kind of theological substance.

Church leaders and historic heroes of the faith were portrayed as having incredible equanimity. I remember stories of faithful martyrs who were killed in various gruesome ways—fed to hungry animals, torn limb from limb, burned to death. Instead of screaming with fear (or feeling any emotion normal humans would in such terrible moments), they smiled forgivingly while singing hymns. Of course, this was a testament to their great faith. It also was an implicit message that really holy people don't feel fear or pain. Or if they do, they don't show it. The people we held up as heroes were calm, collected, solid, and trustworthy. They were never overly emotional, out of control, weak, or afraid.

A RECIPE FOR SICKNESS

I try to talk about the church of my childhood with fairness. Much was good about that community. It's where I met Jesus. It's the school that taught me to love and listen to Scripture. Many faithful, kind followers of Jesus in that community influenced me deeply. But I've had so many conversations with others who shared similar church experiences. Many of us came away from our upbringings believing these myths. The maps we inherited were completely incapable of leading us down the path maturity requires.

If becoming more spiritual means becoming less emotional, we have a serious problem. Emotions happen. They move us. Sometimes they settle into moods or become habitual. While emotions certainly shift, they don't leave us untouched. Grief, fear, or sadness that goes unexpressed stays within us, warping our hearts and relationships. These things don't just go away.

So what happens when you live in a church community like the one I've described? You stop showing emotion. Maybe you even stop feeling emotions. At least you try.

Many people in similar churches who couldn't live this way just left. The rest of us practiced denial, which sounds very spiritual. We'd avoid uncomfortable situations. We'd change the subject. We'd take antacids for the clenching in our guts. Some of us (already on the road to ruin) secretly took antidepressants for our sadness. We treated our negative emotions like the symptoms of a cold, suppressing them with medication, so we could get on with being good Christians.

Not everyone was like this. I knew wonderful, wise, and spiritually mature people in my religious community growing up—even emotionally expressive people—but they always seemed the exception. There were so many more who were immature, emotionally repressed, inflexible, and legalistic. I say this with no bile. Each of these words at one point (sometimes still) described me. It's reasonable to wonder whether the system itself was contributing to the problem.

We talked about God changing us, but that seemed to mean people only stopped smoking, drinking, or sleeping around. It rarely meant they became more kind, more gracious, or more willing to generously serve. We didn't seem to expect that kind of life change.

In the first church I served as a pastor, I encountered an older gentleman I'll call Leonard. Long before I arrived, he had taken charge of the church kitchen. This particular church building had a spectacular commercial kitchen. To use it, you had to go through Leonard. He was brusque and sharp, with a ready lecture at hand. If your group didn't clean up exactly the right way or if, God forbid, you used a piece of equipment without permission, well, let's just say it was going to be a bad day for you. Leonard's angry tirades were familiar, even expected. The day he discovered I'd used the kitchen for a youth-group tie-dye party was a disaster.

This was a problem, because food is always a frequent part of church life. Even more concerning, no one seemed to expect anything different. Leonard had been prickly for as long as anyone could remember. He'd been a member of this church for decades and had been in leadership for years. Everyone accommodated his bad behavior, tiptoeing around his tyranny. No one expected him to grow.

Why would we? Discipleship meant learning more biblical knowledge and theology. Sanctification meant becoming more holy, more morally pure. A good church member was one who served, gave, and showed up. Becoming more whole was just not a part of our plan for spiritual maturity.

These myths about emotions many of us inherited from church are flawed maps. Not only are they wrong; they also lead us away from what is true.

Do emotions always lie? No. Emotions nearly always tell us the truth. It's just not always the truth we think.

Are emotions shallow and transitory? No. Emotions are messages from our deepest places, and they won't just go away if we don't heed them.

Is God unemotional? Unequivocally no. All our emotions were created in God's image. Learning how God is emotional is one of the best ways to understand our own emotions and the guidance they contain.

Will we become less emotional as we grow spiritually? Are emotions sin—something God takes away as we grow? No. In fact, the more connected to God we become and the more spiritually mature we become, the more aware of our emotions and the emotions of others we will be.

Do any of these statements intrigue you? Do they sound different from what you've been taught? In time we'll unpack and support each one. As I flew home to Portland following that pastors' retreat, I was beginning a journey that would lead me, in turn, to each of these truths.

QUESTIONS FOR REFLECTION

1. How would you describe the mental maps about emotions that you gathered and inherited growing up? What did those maps say? Where did they come from?

2. Did you pick up any of the four myths about emotions from your church or religious upbringing? How were these ideas communicated to you? How did they affect you? Were there others?

3. If we never talk about God and emotions, what impact will that inevitably have on our pursuit of becoming more like Jesus?

Part Two

THE UNEXPECTED BIBLE STORY

Chapter 4

THE LOST IMAGE

*How can you love God with your whole
heart, when your heart isn't whole?*
Rick D. Padgett, Westgate Ministries

*Love the Lord your God with all your heart, with
all your soul, with all your strength, and with all
your mind; and your neighbor as yourself.*
Luke 10:27

Flying home from that Minnesota retreat was like entering a new country. Mount Hood still pushed through the clouds, the Columbia River rolling toward the ocean just to the mountain's north. But there was a possibility of something new and better I hadn't felt for as long as I could remember. I had been set on a new path.

Conversations with my counselor friend led me to a decision. It was time to see a therapist. I started by booking a session for marriage counseling. Admitting our marriage needed work was less painful than admitting I needed work. The therapist wasn't fooled. In short order, we began the arduous process of unpacking my story. I needed to understand how I had come to be who I was.

Emotion still felt like a wild, uncontrollable danger. If I could just understand what was happening to me, maybe I wouldn't be so intimidated. I started reading books by people who study emotions—psychologists, emotional theorists, brain researchers, neurosurgeons, and philosophers. I also dug into Scripture. I was growing suspicious that much of what I'd been taught in church about emotion was wrong, but I needed to see for myself. I sought out the reflections of Christian thinkers and theologians, modern and ancient. What I found was unexpected. The Bible was full of emotional language and counsel for this aspect of our lives (which we'll explore in the next two chapters). What's more, there was also a rich historical conversation about the role of emotions in our spiritual lives. I wasn't the only one trying to make sense of this.

For several years I stewed in all these ideas. Of course, what I was learning began to filter into my ministry. I even preached two series of messages about the connection between emotions and following Jesus. I never expected the overwhelming response I got from the congregation. There was hunger, almost a desperate need, to see God in this area of life. I had more emails, private conversations, and feedback regarding these messages about emotion and spiritual growth than anything else I had ever preached on in almost two decades.

WAIT! EMOTIONS IN CHURCH?

A few people wondered aloud why a pastor was taking valuable time to teach about emotions. After all, there is no "book of Emotions" in the Bible. Was I falling off the wagon? Going all psychobabble? I don't think so.

In the gospel of Luke, there's a scene where a religious man approached Jesus with a question: "Teacher, what must I do to inherit eternal life?"

The answer to this question was profoundly important:

> Love the Lord your God with all your heart, with
> all your soul, with all your strength, and with all
> your mind; and your neighbor as yourself.[1]

The most important thing, Jesus said, was to love God with every aspect of our lives—heart, soul, mind, and strength—and our neighbors. Some streams of Christianity have made loving God a matter of right beliefs. Other streams teach that our obedient acts demonstrate our love for God. Each of these perspectives carries part of the truth, but our minds and behavior aren't the whole of us. If we're to love God the way God asks, our love must include more than facts, ideas, and good behavior. Jesus pointed to a kind of love that is heart and soul deep, loving God with our emotions as well. If this is true, then learning about emotions is an important part of learning how to love and follow God.[2]

Being told we must love God with our emotions isn't that helpful, though. It's a bit like when I force my kids to apologize to each other. They enact the forms, but their hearts aren't in it. This is good practice, but we all know the apology isn't the same as one that comes from the heart. We can't be told to *feel* forgiveness. Being told to love God with our emotions is similarly difficult.

The church has, at times, made the task even more complicated. I shared earlier that I grew up in a faith community that
was at best skeptical about emotions. Public displays of emotion
usually meant something was wrong. People could cry when they
repented of their sins, but any other time was suspect. You were
supposed to have faith. Having faith meant not doubting. If you
were feeling doubt or fear, you probably weren't trusting God
enough.

There was also a strong gender bias. Women were emotional.
Men were strong. And strong men didn't show fear or worry. That
meant never losing control. It also meant never crying. All of
this presented a variety of problems for healthy emotional and
spiritual growth. Notice, too, the implied denigration of women.
If emotional expression was a sign of spiritual immaturity, and
if emotions always led you astray, and since it was accepted that
women were more emotional, then it followed that women were
less spiritually mature or trustworthy. Oh, Lord, how much damage did we do?

Not all communities of faith are like mine was, but many are.
It's strange, too, because these churches take the Bible seriously,
yet their view of emotions isn't scriptural.

CAN AN EMOTIONAL CHURCH BE A GOOD THING?

In Romans 12:9–15 (NIV), we find one passage describing what
Christian community can be like:

Love must be sincere. Hate what is evil; cling to what is good. Be devoted to one another in love. Honor one another above yourselves. Never be lacking in zeal, but keep your spiritual fervor, serving the Lord. Be joyful in hope, patient in affliction, faithful in prayer. Share with the Lord's people who are in need. Practice hospitality.

Bless those who persecute you; bless and do not curse. Rejoice with those who rejoice; mourn with those who mourn.

How can you read this passage and wonder whether emotions have any place in church or discipleship? The passage is bursting with emotional energy!

Love sincerely.
Hate evil.
Be devoted.
Never lack zeal.
Have spiritual fervor.
Be joyful, hopeful, patient.
Rejoice with those who rejoice; mourn with those who mourn.

These weren't immature Christians led astray by deceitful emotions. Neither was this a stoic community, growing more serene as they became more like Christ. The community Paul described was experiencing and responding to visceral emotions. Their emotions were part of fully living out the image of God.

Think of all the good (but crazy) choices followers of Jesus sometimes make. Stephanie, a young woman in my church at the time, left a lucrative, secure job to join Wycliffe, the international ministry that translates the Bible into indigenous languages. After just a year of training, she headed off to south Asia to learn one of the languages. Why? So that in a crazy and unexpected way, she might help some people come to know Jesus.

Another family I know invited a homeless couple to live with them for a year. This family radically changed their lifestyle because they felt Jesus calling them to it.

I've also known people who gave beyond their means and others who have offered transcendent forgiveness to someone who violated them.

Why do people do these outrageous acts of kindness and service? It's not just because of duty. It's not only because they have an intellectual understanding of who Jesus is and a philosophical commitment to His values. Scripture and theology influence their thinking, but when it comes down to a costly choice, these people are powerfully moved. Their emotions influence them to act in ways that express the heart of Jesus.

That's what emotions are designed for. They exist to move us. We've all made bad decisions because of our emotions, but what if God's purpose for emotions is just the opposite? What if our emotional and intuitive ways of knowing were given to us to call us forward in goodness, compassion, and love? What if they are in fact access points for the Holy Spirit to move us?

Having had an inside view of people's lives for years, I've come to believe that without spiritually centered emotions, we rarely obey the call of God when it's difficult or inconvenient. Worse, if trauma, training, or habit has muted the voice of emotion in our lives, we may even miss God's voice. I find it sad and ironic that the church has become complicit in distancing us from our emotions. In an effort to be more holy and faithful, we've found ourselves less connected to God and God's guidance.

ONE WRONG INGREDIENT SPOILS THE DOUGH

I walked into the kitchen. My nose told me the truth before I saw the evidence. A fresh batch of cookies was cooling on the counter. Oatmeal raisin—my favorite. I picked one up, ready to savor that delicious blend of spice, sweetness, and butter. The texture was right. The smell was perfect. I bit into the cookie and immediately spat it out. Salt had been mixed into the batter instead of sugar. One ingredient in the recipe was flawed, ruining the entire batch of cookies.

The flawed emotional maps we often inherit from church aren't entirely unexpected. They're a natural result of the recipe used to cook up Christian thought over the centuries. One of the key ingredients was bad, and that has fouled the taste of Christianity in more ways than one.

Starting in the early second century, Christian thinkers, always looking for ways to engage the culture and defend Scripture, began to use ideas and language borrowed from Platonic dualism. By the Middle Ages, Platonic thinking was the accepted description of reality. Greek philosophers, starting with Socrates and his student Plato, taught that everything in the universe, even humanity, exists in two separate states—matter and spirit. Matter was tangible, everything we could see and touch. These material things were manifestations of a larger, greater reality. Spirit was everything we couldn't see, the truth behind the material world. It included our souls and a whole invisible framework behind the universe they called the *logos*.

This worldview had wide-ranging consequences. Spirit was good, true, and everlasting. Matter was transient. It could break, rust, or decay. Matter was just a shadow of what was true, sometimes even a perversion. Our bodies—including bodily processes like hunger, sexual desire, and emotion—were part of the material world. As such, they were looked down on, at times even seen as evil.

Early Christianity grew in the soil of Hebrew culture, with a worldview rooted in the ancient Jewish Scriptures. This worldview was holistic rather than dualistic, but when the church evolved beyond its Hebrew roots into a transnational, transethnic community, theologians were quick to grab onto the intellectual tools of the more cosmopolitan Greeks. As is always the case with any cultural translation, something vital was lost.

The influence of Platonic dualism on the church is hard to overstate. It's a topic far larger than can be discussed here. But know this: most people today, both Christians and non-Christians, believe the Christian view of humanity is dualistic. That's true even for people who have never heard of Platonic dualism.

According to this view, we have bodies and we have souls. They are two separate things. Our bodies are our flesh. They're biological.

They're the vehicles our souls use to get around for the duration of our earthly lives. When this life is over, we will shed our bodies. Only then will our true nature, our souls, be freed. This view sounds like Christian teaching. It's mirrored in popular culture, but this wasn't the early Hebrew view. It may surprise you that this isn't what the scriptural creation story teaches.

WHAT DID GOD MAKE, EXACTLY?

The Genesis creation story says something important about the nature of humanity. Genesis 1 tells the story in a global, cinematic way. Then the camera zooms in, and Genesis 2 tells the same story from a different, grittier perspective. Here God gets dirty fingernails as the first human is formed.[3] The focal point is found in verse 7 (KJV):

> The LORD God formed man of the dust of the ground, and breathed into his nostrils the breath of life; and man became a *living soul.*[4]

God formed humanity from the dust. The word *human* is related to the word *humus*, which means "earth." After forming a body from the tangible matter of earth, God breathed into it the breath of life. That's the moment, the text says, this human "became a living soul." That's the translation in the familiar, old King James. The Hebrew word translated "living soul" is *nephesh*. It can mean "soul," but when you and I hear this word, we're inescapably hearing it through the centuries-old filter of Platonic dualism. In Hebrew, *nephesh* means "living being," "person," or "self." Many modern translations recognize this and translate the phrase "man became a living being." A literal Hebrew reading could be "the human became a self."

Maybe all this sounds like I'm being too picky with words, but this is crucial. The human became a living soul. *Became*. The text doesn't say the human *has* a soul. It says that when God put all the elements of life together, the human *became* a living soul. God created our bodies, all our systems and the tangible parts that make us human. This body had potential, but it lived only with God's breath. Everything we are sprang to life—body, spirit, emotions. At no point in the Genesis story, or anywhere else in the Bible, did God place some sacred little bubble of identity called a soul inside our bodies.

You might not realize the ancient Greek philosophers have shaped your beliefs about emotion. They located the emotions in the body, the fleshly part of us, separate from the spirit. At the least, emotions were distracting hungers. Some philosophers considered them evil influences dragging us away from what was true and spiritual. The church took up this view and has marched on with it ever since.

This Christoplatonism suggests that the soul is the eternal part of you waiting to break the bonds of flesh and sin. Your body is the sweaty, lust-filled, rebellious part of you. As a result, Christian discipleship is often about subjugating, ignoring, or overcoming the flesh. Sound extreme? A few centuries of medieval self-flagellation, another century or two of misguided puritanical preaching, and the "common sense" of countless mothers and pastors are represented in that statement. Our current view that reason is the most elevated part of human consciousness, more trustworthy than emotion, is the modern fruit of this worldview.

However, this bifurcation of our humanity isn't found in the scriptural creation story. Genesis 2 says you *are* your soul and your soul is *all of you*. God created you as a unified being. God made a body for humans from the earth and then breathed life into that body. Your body plus God's gift of life equals a soul.

This has enormous implications for many aspects of Christian discipleship, but for our discussion it means this: your emotions can't be segregated into a corner of your experience. Emotions certainly have to do with your glands and your body, but your body is a part of who God made you to be, and God declared your body and all its systems good. Yes, there are still the fall and the effects of sin. Yes, our bodies are worn and broken. Yes, we need God to restore us! Yet we must never forget that God declared our bodies good.

The Genesis creation story tells us that humanity was created in the image of God. That includes your whole self. There are no verses saying emotions were an afterthought or that they came about as an unfortunate result of sin. No! Your emotions are also made in the image of God, integrated into the fullness of who you are.

This ancient theology mirrors what is now starting to be understood about the body and the brain. For a long time, the brain was seen as a black box, something separate from the body. Some even hypothesized that if you could keep a brain alive in a jar with the necessary sensory inputs wired in, it would still have essential human awareness. Scientists who study these things today are telling a different story. Their studies—the results of new neurological imaging abilities and careful analysis of people with serious brain defects—show that the brain and body are intricately, intimately connected. They aren't separate and unrelated. Unexpectedly, much of the work we've long thought resided in the brain is actually happening all throughout the body. We're learning that our bodies and brains are an integrated whole.

That's what Genesis 2 says too. All of who you are was created in God's image. That means your emotions are made in God's image as well.

WHY TALKING ABOUT EMOTIONS IN CHURCH ISN'T OPTIONAL

There was a second moment of revelation at the Minnesota retreat I attended. We were sitting on folding chairs in a loose circle, discussing pastoral burnout. "Many pastors," Jerry the Therapist said, "are people pleasers. Sometimes because of temperament. Sometimes because of their baggage. They become adept at sensing the emotional needs of their church members. They have to if they want to survive in ministry. Yet, ironically, these same people are often blind to their own emotional reality."

Blind to their own emotional reality? I bristle at being told I don't know things; it's a character flaw. To be told I probably didn't understand my own emotions felt condescending and dismissive. My frustration only grew when Jerry passed out a chart. Like something from elementary school, it listed a few basic emotions—sadness, shame, anger, fear, love, joy, and surprise—with a simple explanation of each.

"This is the emotion of sadness," he began. "Sadness is the emotion we feel when we experience loss." He proceeded through each emotion like this. "This is the emotion of anger. Anger is the emotion we feel when, in our own private logic, we or someone we love has been violated."

I was offended! It felt like a preschool teacher introducing a bunch of unobservant preschool boys to the basic Crayola eight-pack. "Here you go, boys. This crayon is yellow. It's the color of the sun. This one is red. Red is the color of some apples and fire trucks." My rebellious mind was screaming, *I am a grown-up! Don't you think I know all this?*

Later, as I reflected on the day's conversation, it occurred to me that never in my life—not once—had anyone ever sat me down and said anything like this. Not a parent. Not a teacher. Not a pastor. Not a doctor. No one. The conversations my church community had about emotions were few and sounded a single note. I had been told emotions were suspicious. I had been told emotions would cloud my judgment, leading me into sin. I had been told to avoid emotional people, since they weren't dependable. But I had never been told what my emotions meant.

I imagined sitting down with my daughter or son and having that kind of conversation. "Hey, what you're feeling right now, that's sadness. It means you've experienced a loss. That's all. It's not something to be afraid of. It's a feeling, and feelings are the way your brain and body tell you something about an experience you've had. Listen to it. See what you can learn."

This image in my mind rattled me. How would my life have been different if just one person had been able to mentor me in this way? The church I grew up in didn't see emotion as one of God's good gifts. We didn't have a framework for how emotions fit into a life of faith. Nurturing and understanding emotions was just not a part of our plan for discipleship.

Think for a moment about how you envision God. Many hold pictures of God that don't leave room for emotion. God is perfect,[5] but emotions don't feel perfect. God is unchanging,[6] but emotions feel fickle. God makes clear decisions, whereas emotions seem to complicate our choices. This has left many people thinking their only option is a cold, stony God: the unmoved mover, the perfect cosmic Father, distant and judging. Christians can ascribe the soft side to Jesus and the Holy Spirit. Jesus smiles and forgives us. The Holy Spirit gives us warm feelings. But God is hard to relate to—removed, aloof, distant, and implacable.

Surely this must seem like I'm drawing a caricature. But I assure you, in two decades of pastoring, I've seen this picture locked in the minds and hearts of many good people. If your picture of God has any of this in it, even a little, it's a problem. If we believe emotions are merely something to overcome or that spiritual people never have negative emotions, then we set ourselves up for two troublesome obstacles in our relationship with God.

First, we might come to believe the highest expression of our faith is simple duty. Without even noticing, we strip the passion from our lives, trying by force of will to do the right thing just because it's the right thing. Second, we can inadvertently come to think of our relationship with God as little more than an intellectual exercise. Faith becomes no more than a list of doctrines we believe, with passages of Scripture as footnotes.

As a result, we ignore our intuition and emotions as potential avenues of God's guidance. We may end up questioning whether we even have a relationship with God or whether "relationship with God" is just code for agreeing to a list of doctrines. I've met more Christians than I can count who were stuck in this struggle. They do the right things. They believe the right doctrines. They give of their time, talents, and resources. They want to honor God. Yet in a moment of stark vulnerability, they'll admit their life of faith seems hollow. I know this place and its ache so clearly. I've spent so much time there myself. Even as a pastor.

In this place, we don't feel profound joy. We don't feel deeply loved. Our religious life starts to feel like an obligatory to-do list we can never complete. We start wondering, *Maybe I'm doing too much. Maybe I'm burning out. Maybe I need to back off a bit. Maybe those towering New Testament descriptions of the lives of Jesus' followers— caring for one another, meeting regularly, serving the poor, using homes as ministry centers—maybe all of this works only for people who don't have families, jobs, and regular responsibilities.*

Be honest. Am I getting close? Have you sensed this in your own heart? The frustration? The numbness? I've seen them in mine.

We can keep living without a coherent understanding of our emotions, but we'll live reactive lives. As followers of Jesus, we'll be left with little more than dogma or duty. We need an understanding of emotions rooted in Scripture. Why did God create them? How do they reflect God's image? How might sin affect them? What is the Holy Spirit saying through the emotions in our lives? How can we experience them, process them, understand them, and act on them in a way that honors God?

In the book of Ephesians, we find a clear statement of God's purpose for the church:

> He personally gave some to be apostles, some prophets, some evangelists, some pastors and teachers, for the training of the saints in the work of ministry, to build up the body of Christ, until we all reach unity in the faith and in the knowledge of God's Son, growing into a mature man with a stature measured by Christ's fullness.[7]

From God's perspective, the whole purpose of the church is simple: to lead people to maturity.[8] What does this maturity look like? The fullness of Jesus Christ. Let's be clear on this: God's intended purpose for you is to become more like Jesus.

The Genesis creation story says humanity was created in God's image.[9] Sin marred that original, perfect image, but God's work in us and the world is bringing about the eventual and full re-creation of that image. The apostle Paul said in 2 Corinthians 3:18 that we are being transformed into the likeness of Jesus. If our spiritual goal is to become more like Jesus, who is in very nature God, then what we think about God is critically important.

What role did emotion play in Jesus' life? In what way can emotions be said to be a part of God's existence? If we're made in God's image, called to be like Jesus, then that's where we must look next.

QUESTIONS FOR REFLECTION

1. Review Romans 12:9–15, which contains Paul's description of a community of Jesus followers. What emotions do you see Paul describe? What kinds of emotional skills would be needed in a community like this?

2. Have you ever done something good or godly because you were emotionally moved? If so, how was this experience different from times you did the right thing out of duty or simply because it was the right thing to do?

3. Has emotional maturity been a part of discipleship in your life? In what practical ways has your church experience and Christian learning contributed to (or hindered) your emotional health? How could this experience have been different?

Chapter 5

AN EMOTIONAL JESUS?

Jesus Christ is not "only" true God; ... He is a man
like us all, a man without reservation.
He not only resembles us men; He is the same as us.

Karl Barth, *Dogmatics in Outline*

The one who has seen Me has seen the Father.

Jesus (John 14:9)

In a past filled with youth ministry, Vacation Bible School, and summer camps, I've participated in more than my share of fun, weird, and sometimes dubious activities ostensibly intended to teach kids about God. I've seen, even been in, more dramas than I can count, most poorly written and often theologically questionable. Now and again, one of those dramas turned out to be something memorable.

One sketch I still remember presented a sequence of outlandish characters, each one an exaggerated riff on some mistaken view of God. There was the old-time sheriff with a hair-trigger six-shooter and a preoccupation with law and order, the hoary ancient nodding off in his rocking chair between stories about the olden times, and the wishy-washy surfer dude who just wanted everyone to love him. There were other sketches portraying a variety of characters, but I can still see and hear one with crisp recall.

At center stage sat a large cardboard box. It was still for a long beat, leaving the audience wondering. Then my friend Donny would pipe up from inside. In a wavering, anxious voice, he began talking about the religious people who locked God in a box. They liked having God near. They liked telling others God was in their possession, but they never let God out of the box. They didn't want God disrupting their carefully planned worship services. God wanted to fly free, to disturb the self-righteous complacency of people's hearts. The people, however, preferred to keep God locked inside the box. Nearby, but not too near.

The sketch was silly.[1] Donny's squeaky performance of a boxed-up God was absurd. Yet that memory has been a prophetic voice at many points in my life. It was a parable and a warning. How easily I become so committed to my own picture of God. When I do, I lose the ability to be confounded and surprised by God.

We all have pictures of God in mind. Anytime we think about religion or spirituality, our pictures of God become active filters shaping what we think. We may not consider ourselves theologians. Many people even find the words *theology* and *theologian* off-putting. Yet we're all theologians, for we each curate a collection of images of God in our minds.

Fortunately, followers of Jesus have a natural starting point for this discussion. We're not thinking about God in the abstract. We're looking at a person. The apostle Paul tells us that Jesus "is the image of the invisible God."[2] We don't have to wonder what God is like. Like a gardener trimming back overgrown brambles, Jesus came to clear out long-held assumptions about God. "Look at Jesus," we're told. There we see once and for all who God is, how God relates to us, and what we can expect from God. Jesus Himself made this claim: "The one who has seen Me has seen the Father."[3]

WHICH JESUS?

Of course, there's a problem with encouraging people to look at Jesus. Which Jesus are we referring to? All Christians (and many non-Christians) have what they consider to be a well-formed mental picture of Jesus. That picture, however, may draw little from the text that teaches us about Him.

Several paintings and illustrations of Jesus were fixtures in my childhood. These Western portrayals had Jesus looking like some kind of serene spiritual guru, above the struggles of our world. One painting in a childhood picture book portrayed the iconic moment when Jesus scattered the vendors in the temple. All around the edges of the scene, the merchants and temple officials were scrambling to escape, their faces stretched in shock, horror, and fear, as if a bomb had just detonated. In the center of the picture, with an aura of glory surrounding Him, stood Jesus wearing a white robe and blue sash. He was standing strong, like a pillar, a few cords of rope dangling from one hand. His other hand was raised, pointing vaguely stage left, as though He was giving directions.

"Greetings, everyone. Could I just have the merchants gather over here?"

The scrambling merchants were painted with motion and energy, but not Jesus. He was an island of calm holiness installed in the middle of the ruckus.

We often pillory pastors when they get sideways theologically with a misspoken word or a sermon not well thought through. Rarely have we applied the same theological concern to artists. Yet this painting is just so wrong, both historically and theologically.

This moment in the temple was electric. Imagine the tension, the action, if a guest on a White House tour stepped out of the approved route and staged a protest inside the building. Jesus was expelling the money changers the priests had welcomed. He was kicking out the animal vendors the whole sacrificial system depended on. Jesus dangerously violated protocol. This was no serene moment, yet the painting, and a few others like it, portray Jesus in the midst of this wildly subversive act with complete equanimity. No energy. Little visible anger. No zeal.

There are more than a few portrayals of Jesus on the cross with this same interpretive failure. A stylized crown of thorns rests on His brow above a few delicately traced lines of blood. His eyes look out, gazing with detachment. Images like these occupy space in so many of our minds. This Jesus is the product of our imaginations. If we're going to let Jesus inform our emotional lives, we must start with the Jesus we find in Scripture.

WE SHOULD ASK, "HOW DID JESUS FEEL?"

So that's where I turned. I knew I didn't want to overlay some therapeutic construct on top of Scripture. I wanted to hear what Scripture really said. So I began a survey of the Gospels, looking for places where Jesus expressed emotion.

Plenty of passages make it easy to assume that Jesus was acting with emotion. Read about Jesus defending the woman who anointed His feet, and then try imagining this scene without some kind of emotional motivation. It's hard to do. When Jesus rebuked the religious leaders, calling them "whitewashed tombs,"[4] it seems natural that some level of frustration or passion accompanied those words. Yet those are assumptions, a layer of interpretation. My assumptions may be right, but they remain assumptions. That wasn't what I was looking for. I wanted to see *actual emotion* from Jesus recorded in Scripture.

"YES, JESUS LOVES ME"

Thinking of Jesus as loving or compassionate comes easily. This was the Jesus of my childhood. In church we sang "Jesus loves the little children, all the children of the world!" and "Yeeeessss, Jesus loves meeee!" This kind of emotion isn't hard to find in Scripture.

In Mark 10, a rich young man came to Jesus with the central question of religion: "Good Teacher, what must I do to inherit eternal life?" Jesus looked at him and loved him.[5] The word there is *agapao*. This Greek word is translated "love," but we're often taught this is a special, nonemotional love God has for all of us. If that's the case, it makes no sense for the text to point this out. God loves everyone in this way, but the text calls it out specifically. Jesus saw this particular young man, and Jesus loved him even in the middle of his spiritual confusion.

The way the word is used in the story seems more like compassionate fondness than some abstract sacrificial good intention for the young man's best interests. Jesus wasn't responding to the young man because of obligation or because this was a great opportunity to make a point that would eventually become Scripture. Jesus engaged the young man's question because He felt compassion toward him.

This inner motivation of compassion was something Jesus felt repeatedly. Several times in the Gospels, Jesus was moved with compassion. That English phrase comes from one Greek word: *splagchnizomai*. (You pronounce it "splahnk-nee-dzow-my.") What's the meaning of this mouthful? Mercy from the bowels. To be moved in the gut with solidarity and compassion. You see someone in need or in pain, and an urge rises inside you, moving you to act.

Five times this word is used to describe how Jesus saw the crowds following Him. He saw their need and was moved to serve.[6] Three times this word shows up in the text when Jesus was moved to heal someone.[7] Once, Jesus happened across a funeral procession for the only son of a widow. In losing her precious son, she also lost her only source of support and protection in the world. Jesus saw her. Moved with *splagchnizomai*, He stopped the funeral procession and raised the boy from the dead![8]

The three remaining occurrences of this word are fascinating. In each case, Jesus used this word in a story. These three parables don't directly describe Jesus' emotional experience, but they do show Jesus using this powerful word. As He used the word, we gain insight into the kind of experience it described.

In Matthew 18:27, Jesus described a debtor who petitioned his king for relief. The king was moved with compassion to forgive the debt. In Luke 10:33, this word describes the Good Samaritan's motivation to help the injured man lying in the ditch. Finally, in Luke 15:20, Jesus used this word to describe what the father felt when he saw his prodigal son coming down the path toward home.

It's not surprising to find portrayals in Scripture of Jesus being moved with love or compassion. This fits. For Jesus, love was not only a commitment of the will or an orientation of the mind toward humanity. This love was visceral and compelling—a feeling, but not some fluttering, fickle whim. It was a deep, rich experience that moved Him to act.

CAN YOU PICTURE JESUS JUMPING FOR JOY?

Love isn't the only positive emotion Scripture portrays Jesus experiencing. In Luke 10, Jesus sent seventy followers on a mission into the villages of the area. They returned excited. There had been healings and exorcisms. They had seen real kingdom transformation. But they weren't the only ones who were happy.

Luke 10:21 says that when Jesus heard this news, He rejoiced. The word in Greek, *agalliao*, means "to be exceedingly glad." That's dictionary speak for saying that Jesus was giddy. His heart overflowed with joy. People were being transformed, even healed! The root of this word literally means "to leap." It's not inaccurate to say that when He heard this news, Jesus jumped for joy.

Jesus wasn't looking out on the scene with those serene eyes, satisfied in some deep but unemotional way. This was unfettered exultation, happiness visible for everyone to see. You know, real joy!

Seeing Jesus joyful was healing for me. The serene, impassive Jesus of my childhood could be pleased (especially when I obeyed), but this was something better. This was happiness throwing a party.

In fact, happiness throwing a party features in some of Jesus' best-known stories. Luke 15 presents a sequence of parables, each depicting something valuable being lost and then found. Each story culminates in a party—the enthusiastic, communal expression of joy. The woman who found her lost coin and the shepherd who recovered his wandering sheep both gathered their friends for a celebration. When the prodigal son returned, his father was so excited, he threw a huge bash. When Jesus talked about recovering the lost, it evoked a joyful response of celebration.

CAN GOD BE SURPRISED OR SAD?

Surveying the Gospels for moments of emotion in Jesus' life uncovered more than just love, compassion, and joy. There were other emotional experiences, perhaps unexpected for God in the flesh.

In Matthew 8, a Roman centurion came to Jesus. A precious servant was dying, and the officer asked Jesus to heal the man. Jesus offered to go directly to the officer's home, but the Roman refused. He believed Jesus could heal his servant by just saying the word. The text says that Jesus was amazed at the faith of this outsider. Some translations say, "He marveled."[9]

The Greek word here, *thaumazo*, means "to admire, wonder, and be amazed." This word is used more than forty times in the New Testament. When it's used to describe people other than Jesus, it always has an emotional component of surprise and wonder. This word describes the reaction of the disciples when Jesus calmed the storm.[10] It was the reaction of the crowds when Jesus healed people.[11] It showed up when Jesus taught something unprecedented.[12] It was Pilate's reaction when Jesus remained silent at His trial.[13]

This is an experience of wonder and awe. It's hard to imagine God being surprised. The possibility brings up interesting theological questions. Yet here in the text, Jesus had an emotional response of surprise and fascination when He encountered unexpected faith.

That's a wonder, but things get even more complicated. Being God means being powerful, right, and in charge—not a state we associate with sorrow. Yet more than once, Scripture shows Jesus feeling sadness.

Near the end of Luke's gospel, Jesus arrived in Jerusalem to a parade in His honor. The crowds were cheering, hopeful that a new government was about to be put in place. Jesus knew their expectations wouldn't be met. He knew destruction was coming to Jerusalem. As He looked at the city, He wept.[14] Unless His tears were a show, Jesus was feeling grief, crying with profound sadness for the people of Jerusalem.

When His friend Lazarus died, Jesus wept for him too.[15] This wasn't something grand or missional. This was the real pain and grief of losing a loved one to death.

When Jesus' divinity overshadows His humanity in our minds, it pushes Him out of reach. If He were God, He couldn't really be like us, right? How could He ever be surprised or upset? But Jesus was fully human. These passages show us how far "fully" went.

One of the most raw moments of my life happened when I was sitting on a concrete front step, imagining myself driving headlong into the first semitruck I could find. The woman I loved, the woman I hoped to marry, wanted to be with someone else. On that step, pain, white and sharp, punched through my chest, leaving me unable to breathe. My body turned on itself in a fetal hunch, shaking with waves of tears, as if I were in withdrawal.

The pain was so utter, blazing, and dominating. I was desperate for it to stop. In that moment a reckless drive into an oncoming truck made sense. I had enough of myself left to call a friend. I can't imagine what he heard in my inarticulate cry for help, but he talked me through that crushing moment and got me safely home.

Grief is so naked, so vulnerable, so unlike God, we think. Yet Scripture shows Jesus experiencing this very emotion, multiplied beyond understanding. The garden of Gethsemane was the scene, God's concrete front step, tense with emotional energy, pain, and fear. It's humbling, almost embarrassing, to read. If I were constructing the story of a spiritual hero, I would never include such raw details. In the garden, Jesus collapsed in agony. He begged His friends to sit with Him, to give Him comfort. The impending torture of body and spirit was overwhelming.

In Mark's gospel, this anguish is expressed in Jesus' words: "My soul is swallowed up in sorrow—to the point of death."[16] This is sadness so deep, so visceral, it's experienced as physical pain. My pain from being rejected was a tiny fleck, a shard, of what Jesus experienced. Still, His words make perfect sense to me. To know that God-in-the-flesh felt racking grief and pain, to know that my deepest moments of vulnerability aren't outside God's experience, this cracked open my picture of God, flooding it with grace. It was like discovering a vast valley of emotional depth illuminated by the lightning strike of Gethsemane.

CAN GOD FEEL "UNGODLY" EMOTIONS?

Sadness isn't the only difficult emotion the Gospels portray Jesus experiencing. There are others that push beyond the boundaries of what seems acceptable.

We've already talked briefly about the powerful scene when Jesus cleared the temple courts. This moment is debated among biblical scholars. Some argue it was a teaching moment, a living parable of divine justice. Others point to it as a tangible expression of God's wrath manifested in the person of Jesus. Some commentators go to enormous lengths to make clear that Jesus was in control during this whole episode, measured in His actions. In fact, they argue, Jesus was defending decorum and civility.[17] It's uncomfortable for some to picture Jesus as just plain angry.

The gospel of John was written with the benefit of the most time and reflection after this event. John showed the disciples remembering Jesus' actions in the temple courts as the fulfillment of an Old Testament prophecy.[18] The verse they remembered? Psalm 69:9: "Zeal for Your house has consumed me." Zeal. Today that word often means a nice, clean, righteous energy, but the Greek word, *zelos*, is raw. It's a burning, fierce indignation, even jealousy. This is the pot boiling over.

Jesus was indignant because people were being priced out of worship. He was jealous for the holiness—the set-apartness—of the sanctuary. He was filled with fury that the machinery of the temple system had turned a house of prayer, meant for people to come near to God, into a gated community keeping them out. Maybe Jesus was making a theological point, but He sure was doing it emotionally.

In Mark 8:11, some cynical religious leaders asked Jesus to perform a sign. They wanted Jesus to prove Himself or perhaps to provide something they could use to discredit Him. Verse 12 says, "Sighing deeply in His spirit, He said, 'Why does this generation demand a sign?'"

Sighing deeply in His spirit. You know the feeling, the groan of frustration when you can't believe what you're hearing. Maybe your kids blithely do what you've told them a hundred times not to do, or your boss emails the whole office at four thirty, announcing that everyone has to work late today. That's frustration, and frustration is anger behaving politely.

Another time, a gaggle of children wanted to see Jesus. His disciples felt that Jesus was too important to be spending His time this way. They shushed the children, sending them away. Jesus' response? "He was indignant and said to [His disciples], 'Let the little children come to Me.'"[19] Jesus was indignant. That's another kind of anger. The Greek word means "greatly afflicted."

IF WE'VE SEEN JESUS …

For Christians, the starting point for thinking about both God and emotions is Jesus. If Jesus is our model, then we can safely say that anything we see in the life of Jesus can have a healthy, even godly, place in our own lives. But Jesus isn't simply a model to follow; He is the incarnation of God. "The one who has seen Me has seen the Father," Jesus said.[20] When we look at Jesus, we see what we need to know about God. If we think we know something about God and it doesn't square with Jesus and His teaching, then we're wrong. This is the epicenter of all our theology—including our thoughts about emotion and faith. Everything moves out from there.

What have we seen? Jesus wept for Lazarus. He felt anguish over Jerusalem. He felt crushing loneliness and grief in the garden. He longed for friends who would sit with Him in His pain. He was frustrated when religious leaders demanded a sign, indignant when His friends tried to keep children away from Him. Jesus even got angry—flipping-over-the-tables angry—with the leaders who were obstructing the people's path to God. Jesus celebrated, maybe even jumped for joy, when His disciples returned from their first successful mission.

Let these scenes of Jesus' emotions play in your mind, and then consider this: Scripture teaches that Jesus is the "exact representation"[21] the "[visible] image of the invisible God."[22] It also says Jesus never sinned.[23] Yet He got angry. He was sad. He expressed painful feelings. Do you see how this changes things? If all of this is true, it means that none of these emotional expressions are sinful. None were deficiencies in Jesus' character or demonstrations of emotional or spiritual immaturity. More importantly, this means those emotions are part of God's experience too.

QUESTIONS FOR REFLECTION

1. Think back on the picture of Jesus you've had in the past. How would you describe His emotional life? What kinds of emotions did you expect Jesus to feel?

2. Positive feelings such as joy, compassion, and love seem to fit neatly into our picture of Jesus. Yet Scripture shows Jesus also experiencing emotions we're far less comfortable with, such as anger and grief. How does seeing this affect your view of Jesus?

3. The incarnation means that Jesus was both fully God and fully human. It's easy to ascribe all the emotions we discussed to Jesus' human side, yet He told us, "If you've seen Me, you've seen the Father." What do Jesus' emotions tell us about God?

4. Does thinking about Jesus' emotions cause you to rethink your theology in any way? How so?

Chapter 6

AN UNCOMFORTABLY MESSY PICTURE OF GOD

To love at all is to be vulnerable.

C. S. Lewis, *The Four Loves*

God is love.

1 John 4:8

I grew up on the story of Jesus. Scenes of His life are iconic in my memory: cleansing the temple, restoring life to a little girl at her father's request, defending the woman accused of adultery, teaching Nicodemus late at night, and welcoming the little children. Of course, there were also the troubling scenes of Passion Week—experiencing that painful night in the garden, begging the Father for relief, stumbling under the weight of the cross, enduring the beatings and the crucifixion, and then forgiving those who hurt Him.

These images and so many others are clear in my mind, gritty in detail. It wasn't hard for me to get on board with Jesus having emotions. He had a body, after all, with the same glands and neuro-transmitters you and I have. He had experiences and responded to them. Even being perfect and holy, at the least He would understand what I felt.

But making the leap from Jesus to God, the omnipotent creator and ruler of the universe? Considering the emotions of the Father? That was a stretch. I've learned I'm not alone in this.

SO MANY MISGUIDED IMPRESSIONS

What image comes to mind when you picture God? This time, I'm not talking about Jesus.[1] I'm not asking about your theological explanations for the nature and qualities of God the Father. I'm asking about the immediate mental image you most associate with God. Got it? With that image in mind, ask yourself this question: What do you think God's emotions are like?

I've asked many people this question, even people who aren't Christians. Among people who think there is a God, I've found remarkable consistency in the answers.

Some people think God is predominantly angry, full of judgment. The world is so broken, with people relentlessly hurting one another. How could God not be angry?

Others think God is only loving. When pressed about what this means, they often can't bring themselves to say they view it as an emotional love. They describe God as having benevolence toward everyone, forgiving anyone who asks. Rarely do they describe this love in feeling terms. They think of love as a divine attribute. Water is wet; God is love.

The most common response people give by far is that they never even considered God as having emotions. Perhaps God has qualities that share the same name as our emotions. God is love. God expresses wrath. But they don't picture those as visceral, motivational feelings. Emotions seem so human—unpredictable, fickle, untrustworthy. God isn't like that, so God must not have emotions.

So which is it? Angry? Loving as an attribute but not as an emotion? Unemotional? These responses tell us more about our discomfort with emotions than they do about God. They also highlight that our mental images of God often have little to do with Scripture. God as the angry bearded old man depends more on classical representations of Zeus than it does on the descriptions offered in Jewish and Christian Scriptures. The vague image of God as the unmoved mover, sustaining the universe but with no personal connection to us, is constructed from the raw materials of Greek philosophy. They're familiar images, but none speak accurately of the God portrayed in the Bible.

If we're created in God's image and God designed our emotions with a purpose, then we must look past the assumptions we carry. If a survey of the Gospels showed us things about Jesus we didn't expect, might it be the same when we look past the layers of interpretation we inherited to understand the heart of God?

In the same way I reviewed the Gospels, looking for indications of emotions in Jesus' life, I turned to the rest of Scripture, searching for descriptions of emotions in God's experience. I didn't have to look far. The chronicle of God's emotions starts at the beginning of the story and runs through the last pages. The depth and variety of emotion in God's experience surprised me.

IF YOU CAN PLEASE GOD, GOD CAN EXPERIENCE PLEASURE

Can God experience pleasure? The Genesis creation story shows God feeling satisfaction. Repeatedly we hear, "God saw that it was good."[2] Like any artist, God took pleasure in the work of creating. When God offered to give King Solomon anything he desired and then Solomon asked for wisdom, God was pleased.[3] Colossians 1:19 says God was pleased to have all the fullness of divinity dwell in Jesus. Hebrews 13:16 tells us that when we sacrificially share with others, it brings pleasure to God. We also see that God was pleased at Jesus' baptism. The way Matthew tells it, when Jesus came out of the water, the heavens parted and God spoke: "This is my Son, whom I love; with him I am well pleased."[4] The Greek word means "to take great pleasure in." This isn't a declaration of intellectual approval; it's an emotional response to something good and right.

God's pleasure in Scripture runs even deeper than this. God experiences delight, that heart-lifting combination of pleasure and joy. In the ancient book of Zephaniah is a song of encouragement and hope for the daughter of Zion, culminating in one of the most precious images in Scripture:

> Yahweh your God is among you,
> a warrior who saves.
> He will rejoice over you with gladness.
> He will bring you quietness with His love.
> He will delight in you with shouts of joy.[5]

Here is God, the creator and king of the universe, looking at a daughter hard pressed when facing her enemies and difficult circumstances. Seeing her, God is deeply moved. The New International Version renders that last line "[He] will rejoice over you with singing." The Hebrew is a jumble of emotions, with words that can mean joy, rejoicing, singing, mirth, exultation, and shouting. God is so happy to see this daughter, the only natural response is to dance and sing!

Sure, this is a song, and artists use extravagant language. God is spirit, and spirits don't have legs, so there's surely not dancing involved in the traditional sense. Yet no matter how you interpret these lines, this is clearly not just some muted intellectual benevolence. This is exuberant, spontaneous elation. With this kind of feeling, God must profoundly care for us.

THE EMOTION AT THE HEART OF GOD'S HEART

Scripture also frequently shows God experiencing compassion. In Hosea 11:8, God was speaking of Israel in the midst of rebellion. The people had wandered so far away that God used the metaphor of a wife who left home to have sex with strangers. Consequences were rearing up, and God saw what was coming:

How can I give you up, Ephraim?
How can I surrender you, Israel?
How can I make you like Admah?
How can I treat you like Zeboiim?

> I have had a change of heart;
>
> My compassion is stirred!

The people abandoned their commitment; they deserved God's judgment. Yet compassion moved God's heart. That's the essence of emotion.

Second Kings 13:23, in the midst of an account of the terrible kings of Israel and how Israel violated the covenant, points out that God didn't disown or destroy the people. Why? Because of compassion. Nehemiah 9:19 tells us that because of compassion, God didn't abandon the Israelites in the wilderness, despite their idolatry. Isaiah 49:13 suggests that one reason we should celebrate is the frequency with which God shows compassion. Compassion isn't an alien or infrequent experience for God; it's ongoing.

Of course, compassion is a sibling of the most vital, vibrant emotional experience—love. Jesus is loving; that's what we learned growing up. All the songs say so. But let's be clear: Jesus is loving because love is the heart of God. Interpret this love as a mere attribute, an abstract benevolence, and we miss one of the most life-giving messages of Scripture. God *is* love, yes, but God also experiences love and expresses love for us!

The most obvious verse to confirm this is also the most famous verse in the Bible, John 3:16 (NIV): "For God so loved the world that he gave his one and only Son." Not only does this verse tell us God feels love; it also portrays how emotions work. We'll talk more about this later, but look closely at the sequence. An object inspired God's love: the world. Seeing the plight of the people in the world evoked love in God's heart. That love wasn't an abstract idea. It moved God to act. The reason Jesus came—the reason we have Jesus as a window into God's heart—is nothing other than love. The same love that precipitated the incarnation is the love that has moved every act of God in human history.

This isn't just a New Testament thing. Long before Jesus showed up, the prophet Jeremiah gave us God's words: "I have loved you with an everlasting love; I have drawn you with unfailing kindness."[6] The Hebrew word here is *hesed*. "Unfailing kindness" is such a weak translation, but *hesed* is no weak word. It's tough to translate because there is no direct English equivalent. *Hesed* contains elements of loyalty, mercy, and compassion, and it always includes action. *Hesed* is rooted in commitment, even covenant. It simply doesn't exist without a tangible expression. *Hesed* describes the entirety of the experience of other-centered loving.

The Old Testament is cut through with this word. It appears nearly 250 times. It describes God's generosity in saving Lot,[7] God's favor in sustaining Joseph in prison,[8] and the motivation for God's stunning rescue of the Israelites in Exodus.[9] Over and over, this word is presented as one of God's core qualities.[10] Some scholars suggest that *hesed* is the biblical concept the New Testament writers were thinking of when they co-opted the Greek word *agape,* using it to define a committed, other-centered, self-sacrificial love leading to action in the world.

This is the love God has for us. This kind of love motivated God to act, to rescue, and to redeem. This love kept God working among humanity in spite of sin, rebellion, and distraction. It laid the foundation for a covenant that remained strong even when people did not. God loves all of us "with a Never Stopping, Never Giving Up, Unbreaking, Always and Forever Love."[11]

Scripture repeatedly describes God in emotional terms. It seems this is the image God wants us to have. God is introduced several times in the Old Testament, and each time the introduction is similar. The words chosen aren't the ones you'd expect to describe divinity. Exodus 34:6–7 is one example:

> Yahweh—Yahweh is a compassionate and gracious God, slow to anger and rich in faithful love and truth, maintaining faithful love to a thousand generations, forgiving wrongdoing, rebellion, and sin.

How many of these qualities are emotional expressions? God is compassionate. God is gracious. God is slow to respond in anger. God is gushing with so much *hesed* that it overflows in forgiveness, even limiting the scope of consequences. This is a God who has chosen to be defined by emotions.

THEN THINGS GET SCARY

Joy, delight, compassion, and love are wonderful, but those aren't our only emotions. Neither are they the only emotions Scripture ascribes to God. If we read the Bible without avoiding the difficult parts, we can't escape this conclusion: God even has emotions that make us feel uncomfortable.

Right about now, you may be sensing a growing discomfort. Your mind may already be putting the pieces together. A voice inside may be saying, *See, this is why God can't have emotions!* You know the weight sadness, anger, wrath, and even hatred can carry. You know how easily they undo you, bringing out your worst. That can't happen to God, right? The line between those emotions and sin seems so blurry. How could a perfect God have anything to do with feelings that seem dark and difficult?

These are fair questions. Before we address them, just notice whatever discomfort you're feeling. Perhaps anxiety is surfacing. Or maybe you're experiencing a creeping sense of boredom, not aware that this mental coping mechanism blunts our thoughts when we touch on emotionally disruptive topics. Your discomfort could also be appearing in the form of intellectual arguments. Perhaps theological or scriptural arguments are coming into your conscious thoughts, suggesting all of this isn't even worth listening to. You might even feel a touch of anger if you sense a challenge to deeply held beliefs. Your emotional response may manifest as feelings, as body sensations, as unbidden thoughts, or even as an inability to think clearly.

The idea that God has emotions is a big stretch for many. Even further, the idea that God might be familiar with some of our most painful and dark emotions just seems, well, heretical. Yet there is something vital here to consider.

GOD IN THE WHIRLING STORM OF DIFFICULT EMOTIONS?

Terrible, painful emotion has marked the worst moments in my life. I felt a panicked uncertainty when my closest fourth-grade friends excluded me from a birthday game, laughing at my confusion. As an adult, I experienced the searing pain of sadness when the woman I loved chose someone else over me. I remember the desolation that settled in my heart when my dad died. I still wrestle with a dark, infectious hatred that wound around my heart when a close friend was brutally beaten and permanently injured by people in trusted positions of authority. Could God possibly know or have experience with emotions like these?

You don't have to wait long in the biblical narrative to come across the answer. Scripture frankly and unapologetically shows God experiencing some of the emotions we find hard or painful.

In Genesis 6, God saw the downward spiral of humanity awash in pride, hatred, and oppression. The text says that God regretted making humanity. God was "grieved in His heart."[12] The Hebrew word means "to be in pain, to be vexed, to be tortured." God's children were hurting one another, twisting and desecrating the divine image within them. God's response? Grief, the painful emotion we feel when something we care about is lost.

Scripture repeatedly makes this claim: God can be moved to feel grief. This is a God whose very heart is accessible and vulnerable. What can cause such a tremor in the divine heart? You and I!

Ephesians 4 says we have the ability to affect God emotionally. "Don't grieve God's Holy Spirit,"[13] we're warned. The Greek word *lupeo* means "to affect with sadness." This is the same word used to describe the young man who left in sorrow because Jesus had told him to give away all his possessions.[14] It's also the word used to describe Jesus' sorrow in the garden of Gethsemane.[15] This isn't a literary device to warn us away from sinful behavior.[16] It's a visceral experience of the emotion of sadness. It's astonishing to consider. We can evoke this feeling in God's heart!

Perhaps sadness seems like an acceptable emotion for God. If God is Father and we are children, God must experience grief when we're hurt or hurt others. Human history is a never-ending parade of oppression and destruction. If God loves us so deeply, then God's heart must never stop hurting. But other emotions stretch and challenge our view of God.

Moses recited the story of Israel's wanderings in Deuteronomy 1. In this narrative, he pointed out that God heard the people's unbelief and became furious with them.[17] Furious! Just a few verses later, with the kind of honesty we wish all leaders shared, Moses admitted that God was angry with him personally. Moses and the people chose not to trust God. In response, God felt anger. That's the emotion we feel when something or someone we love is threatened.

Sometimes God's anger is a response to human choices. Sometimes it's connected to actions of judgment.[18] Jeremiah 30:24 says, "The LORD's burning anger will not turn back until He has completely fulfilled the purposes of His heart." This anger is powerful and dangerous, a consuming fire.[19]

Sometimes God's anger is connected with jealousy. Exodus 34:14 is one of many passages that tell us God is jealous. This is deep water. *Jealousy* is a bad word in our culture. We think of jealous people as insecure, controlling, and unhealthy. Yet God is not only portrayed in Scripture as jealous; God also self-identifies as "a jealous God."[20]

Because anger is the emotion we feel when something we love is threatened, it's often tied in with jealousy. Both of these emotions can also escalate into hatred. For some, the idea that God feels hate is simply not okay. Again and again I've heard people say, "That's why I don't read the Old Testament. I believe in a God of love." Yet Scripture tells us there are things God hates.

Proverbs 6 lists seven things God hates—arrogant eyes, lying tongues, the hurting of innocents, wicked scheming, the rush to do evil, false witnesses, and those who stir up discord in community.[21] Deuteronomy 12:31 says God hates child sacrifice (good thing!). Psalm 5:6 says God hates people of "bloodshed and treachery." Psalm 11:5 says God hates those who love violence. Apparently, God also hates religious feasts and holidays not backed up with loving behavior.[22] Throughout the Old Testament, we repeatedly see God hate idolatry in the same way a loving spouse hates infidelity. God also hates pride, since it thwarts an individual's ability to grow or have an intimate relationship (with God or anyone else). God hates violence, injustice, deception, contentiousness, and insincere worship.

If inner alarm bells are triggering anxiety for you, let me ease your concern. In the next section of this book, we'll talk about all these dark emotions again, looking at how they are rooted in God's love. For now, consider that our anxiety around anger, jealousy, and hatred comes from our experience of broken people reacting to these emotions in destructive ways. That's something we need not fear with God. Where these words show up in Scripture, we find important clues for understanding God's love and what God wants for us. In God, these emotions have a loving and redemptive purpose.

CAN WE HANDLE A GOD WITH EMOTIONS?

Consider the range of God's emotions portrayed in the Bible. It's remarkable, isn't it? God chooses to be identified by emotional language. Over and over Scripture declares God's emotional response to us, to our choices, to our circumstances. Not only does God know and feel the full range of positive emotions, but God is also familiar with heavy, painful emotions, the ones that can undo us. The picture Scripture paints of God is messy, with rough edges, quite unlike the pristine, unmoved mover so many of us have imagined. This can be an uncomfortable realization, yet perhaps it's an improvement over our old pictures of God.

I love the kitchen nook in our home. A round white table sits in a small alcove next to three windows looking down on a front yard shaded by an enormous, ancient Japanese maple. When the table is clear and I'm the only one home sitting there with my laptop and a cup of Earl Grey, sunlight streaming in, this is one of my favorite places in the world.

Most of the time, though, the table isn't clear. Because it's near the front door, the kitchen nook is unavoidably the most convenient place to drop our piles when we come home. Most days, the white table is layered with mail, homework, receipts, and art projects, all flowing around bowls crusted with breakfast remains.

Some days the clutter frustrates me. It confounds my desire for the world to be well ordered. But mostly, it desecrates the image I have in my mind of the perfect, undistracted writing spot. Other days I can see a different perspective. The white table is the epicenter of my family's life; the interwoven layers are artifacts of this season in our lives. The license renewal for our camper came in the mail. That secondhand camper carries fun summer memories. There are receipts from a recent grocery trip, a reminder of God's provision carrying us through a tight financial time. Scattered among the piles is a collection of magnetic building toys, my son's current fascination. The top layer is a fan of homework sheets covered in my daughter's developing handwriting. She's been working so hard lately, but not so hard she can't draw pictures of all the animals she's planning to own in her future life as a dancing veterinarian YouTuber.

Is all this clutter getting in the way of the pure and perfect? Or is it an honest representation of the many good facets giving my life contour and character? Perhaps the piles are pure and perfect in a better way. I have the opportunity to decide how I see.

With Scripture, we have a similar opportunity. The Bible is unquestionably rich with emotional descriptions of God. For some of us, this language is uncomfortable. These emotions carry baggage we'd rather not associate with God. We immediately want to distance ourselves from this messy reality with theology and philosophy. The pure, untouched ideal is comfortable, but what if that emotional language is important? What if it is an honest description of the contour and character of the One in whose image we were made? Perhaps what seems messy is, in fact, the best, truest picture we have of God.

QUESTIONS FOR REFLECTION

1. Before reading this chapter, how would you say you imagined God's emotional life?

2. Reread Exodus 34:6–7, where God is introduced. The language in this introduction is stunningly emotional. Why do you think God would choose to be identified in this way?

3. Many believe in a passionless God, the unmoved mover. But Scripture clearly shows God being moved. Does this change your view of God? How might this emotional language referring to God affect your spiritual life?

4. This chapter and the previous one deal with our mental pictures of God. How might these ideas about God bear practical fruit in your life and relationships with others?

Chapter 7

THE BREATHTAKING AFFECTIONS OF AN INFINITE HEART

There's a wideness in God's mercy I cannot find in my own, and He keeps His fire burning to melt this heart of stone, keeps me aching with a yearning, keeps me glad to have been caught in the reckless, raging fury that they call the love of God.

Rich Mullins, "The Love of God"

My thoughts are not your thoughts, and your ways are not My ways.... For as heaven is higher than earth, so My ways are higher than your ways, and My thoughts than your thoughts.

Isaiah 55:8–9

Our picture of God is central to how we understand and do life, including our emotional lives. Far from being abstract or academic theology, this is vital for a growing, vibrant spiritual life. That's why I want to address two arguments against God having an emotional life.

When I read the Bible, specifically paying attention to emotional language, I was overwhelmed by the roller coaster of emotion from page to page. We see the emotions of sinful people, certainly. We also see desperate, oppressed people emotionally calling out to God. We see emotion in the lives of heroes, leaders, and apostles. All this human emotion happens against the backdrop of God's emotions pouring out across time—powerful, compelling, sometimes confusing, even intimidating.

If you're an emotional person, realizing this may be of enormous encouragement to you. Your life experience isn't an anomaly, outside the range of what it means to be a "good Christian." But for many raised in a Western, rationalist culture, it's not encouraging. It may even be frightening. Isn't emotion at the root of extremist fundamentalism and all the violence it has brought into our world? Aren't the stories of God's anger and wrath just fodder for those who want to demonize their enemies?

Many biblical interpreters seem committed to avoiding these questions. When they encounter emotional language in Scripture, they spiritualize it. I've heard sermons suggesting joy in the Bible is most certainly not an emotion but instead some special theological state. It's not something you feel but something you choose, or something God anoints you with. When it comes to the difficult emotions of God, a common response is that this emotional language is just anthropomorphic, taking a human quality and ascribing it to God to make a point. God doesn't really hate. It's just a literary expression of God's extreme disapproval. God's not really jealous. That's just a strong word so we can understand how important our relationship with God is.

Picturing God with emotions can be difficult for some of us. From certain theological perspectives, it's a contradiction. If God has emotions, especially the painful ones, what does that mean? How does this align with the idea that God never changes?

ISN'T GOD UNCHANGING?

Here is the first critique. God doesn't change; therefore, emotions can't affect God. Theologians call this the impassability of God, a doctrine that God isn't subject to or governed by passions. Scriptures like Malachi 3:6,[1] Numbers 23:19,[2] and James 1:17[3] provide biblical support for this view. God's impassability seems important for practical reasons. If God flip-flops as feelings shift, that doesn't seem safe. It's not predictable. It's not even loving!

But those few Scripture passages stand in contrast to vastly more, suggesting that God is affected in some way by us and the world. Our sin cannot make God grieve if God is impassable. The negotiations between Abraham and God regarding Sodom,[4] and later between Moses and God over the Israelites' sin,[5] make no sense if God isn't open to hearing from us and responding. Through the Old Testament prophets, God repeatedly offered if-then promises. Judgment and consequences were coming as a result of sin. But if God's people would turn away from idols and return to righteousness and justice, then God would relent and show mercy. These promises were simply not truthful if there is no potential for God to adjust a course of action.[6]

I suspect the doctrine of impassability is less about biblical theology and more about our own fear and uncertainty. When we feel anger, hate, or jealousy, that emotion can overpower us. We find ourselves acting in ways that don't reflect who we want to be. When we're angry, most of us can't also be fair. When we hate, we can't also be merciful. When we feel jealousy, it's not usually rightful.[7] We have little experience of these emotions as expressions of love.

Our assumption is that if God experiences these emotions, God would be affected as we are. That seems scary. It also seems to violate scriptural statements about the character of God. But here we run the risk of making God in our own image, assuming that since we've never seen anger expressed lovingly or have never experienced righteous jealousy, they must not exist. Our assumption isn't logical.

For our own emotional safety, we box up God in an intellectual framework with no room for divine emotion. When we do this, we aren't being faithful to Scripture. There simply is no passage in the Bible suggesting that emotional language should be interpreted only metaphorically. The Bible writers themselves seemed stubbornly committed to the idea that these emotions are real. As best as I can tell, the only reason this interpretation is popular is because it's safe. It allows us to spiritualize away Scripture that seems complicated, even frightening.

AREN'T THESE EMOTIONAL WORDS JUST A LITERARY DEVICE?

The second critique grows from the first. If we accept the impassability of God as truth, then we must deal with all that emotional language in the Bible. The way commentators most often do this is to suggest these references are just examples of anthropomorphism—a literary device used to describe nonhuman objects using human imagery.[8] To say "the sunset was happy and welcoming" isn't literally true. Sunsets can't smile. They have no capacity to extend welcome or consider us in any way.

There's no question the Bible is full of anthropomorphisms. Psalm 89:13 is one verse of nearly seventy mentioning God's "right hand." In various verses, God has a strong right hand, a right hand full of righteousness, or a right hand providing victory. But God is spirit; God doesn't actually have a hand. That's just a metaphor for God's strength and ability to act. Isn't it fair, then, to assume that emotional words describing God are also metaphorical?

The Bible describes God as spirit, invisible with no physical form. So when Scripture says God has a strong right hand, that must be a metaphor, but there is no equivalent passage telling us God has no emotions. This argument isn't based on Scripture at all. It's based on philosophical preconceptions rooted in Aristotelian ideals and Platonic dualism, fortified by our own discomfort with emotions.

At first it may seem wise to suggest that when Scripture tells us God is angry or jealous, this is only a metaphor. That's certainly more comfortable, especially for those of us who have experienced abuse or pain at the hands of angry or jealous people. But consider what this would mean. If God's anger is a metaphor, so then is God's compassion. If God's jealousy is a metaphor, so too is God's love.

Love. Passion. Mercy. Delight. These are all emotions. To suggest they are some kind of theological abstraction, simple anthropomorphisms, strips them of any power. To say God celebrates with joy is meaningless if it's not describing a surge of pleasure. To suggest God's love is a cerebral state of benevolence aimed in our direction is to simply gut the concept. This kind of doctrinal love is left with no potency, no ability to transform.

When we talk about God, of course, all our words are incomplete. We must speak in metaphors. How else could we talk about a being so far beyond us? Yet in a way that's hard to fully comprehend, God's emotions aren't metaphorical. The Bible portrays God as emotional not because we're projecting our own thoughts onto God but because God has chosen to reveal this about the divine nature.

In Scripture, God experiences emotions, and we are made in God's image. That means our emotions are also made in God's image. That's why we feel. Certainly sin, pride, and painful personal experiences corrupt our emotions, but even in our best state, we still feel.

WHAT AN INFINITE HEART CAN DO

Instead of the impassibility of God, defended by the interpretive tool of anthropomorphism, we need something more robust. Most Christians, most theists for that matter, hold to three classical definitions of the attributes of God. Theologians and philosophers refer to these ideas as "the three omnis": omnipotence, omniscience, and omnipresence.[9]

Omnipotence is the idea that God is big enough to contain and wield all power. *Omniscience* suggests that God is big enough to contain and comprehend all knowledge. *Omnipresence* is the belief that God is big enough to be everywhere at once. That's a big God. Nothing is more powerful. There is no knowledge beyond this mind, no place out of reach. There is no experience beyond God.

If all of this is true, there's something else we ought to consider: if God is big enough to know all things, God is also big enough to contain and experience all emotions. Perhaps we should add a new word to the collection. God is *omnimotive.*

For humans, emotions are rooted in the body, a composite experience of chemicals, electrical signals, body posture, and the meaning-making of our minds. Omniscience would allow God to understand these feelings without needing a body. Omnipresence means that God has witnessed and experienced every kind of emotionally reactive situation. Omnipotence creates the possibility for God to feel any emotion without the negative impact we experience. Strong emotions can derail us, surprise us, even undo our deepest commitments, but perhaps this isn't an inherent quality of emotion. Maybe it's a limitation of being human.

Our discomfort with an emotional God is a projection of our fears and the limitations we place on God. We're the creatures who have inherent limitations because of our nature, our bodies, the world we live in, and even the effects of sin. God isn't limited in those ways. In the same way God has an infinite mind, infinite presence, and infinite power, God also has an infinite heart. For an infinite heart, emotions are something different. Unlike us, God isn't absorbed in pride. Anger doesn't cause God to lose control. Grief doesn't overwhelm God's capacity to think. God is always God, only, always, and ever love.

So while emotions don't have the power to change God's character, God's emotions are so far beyond ours in terms of depth and potency, we can't even imagine them. We see injustice in the world. For some, it's regrettable. For others, it causes deep personal pain, especially if we've had similar experiences. But when God sees injustice, the sadness and anger God feels are so vast that if we were to experience a fraction of these emotions, we would be crushed. When God experiences joy and satisfaction, the fullness of those feelings is the size of the universe. The most wonderful experience you can imagine would be bland and meaningless in comparison.

Because God has an infinite mind, infinite power, and an infinite heart, emotions don't disrupt God's character. They don't move God to act in ways that are anything other than ultimately loving. We have nothing to fear, for all of God's emotions ultimately flow from God's love.

A GIFT, NOT A CURSE

When I started my study of emotions in the Bible, I didn't know what I'd find. The maps I carried with me suggested emotions were a weakness, markers of spiritual immaturity, something to manage and overcome. But I didn't find a scriptural concession to human emotion, offering God's grace for one more failure. I found a full-hearted embrace of our emotional lives.

The Scriptures drip with emotional language. Figures like Moses, Deborah, Joseph, Mary, Peter, and Paul all showed and acted on emotion. They weren't condemned for it. Jesus Himself showed a rich emotional life. Why wouldn't He? His emotions were the expression of neurological and physiological responses common to all humans, natural processes God designed.

The Bible simply doesn't support the idea that emotions are a result of the fall or a negligible bodily function we'll shed when we get to heaven. We have emotions because we were created in the image of God. Someone might argue that emotions are just the result of chemicals and electricity—bodily functions God doesn't have. True, but consider that God is the one who designed and created those processes. In our amazing bodies, God created an organic system that gives us the same kinds of experiences God has, but on a scale appropriate to humanity.

With emotions, God gave us a gift, not a curse, a small reflection of God's own experience. God gave us the ability to know in a way that runs deeper than our rational understanding, an ability to sense truth in ourselves, in our relationships, and in the world around us. That is the gift of wisdom.

You have emotions because God made you that way. God made you that way because emotions are also part of God's experience. Emotions aren't a glandular legacy of our evolutionary past. Emotions aren't the result of psychological baggage that needs healing. Emotions aren't sin. Emotions are an integral part of who you were made to be.

That old image of God as inaccessible and unmoved isn't the Father of Jesus Christ. If our goal is to mature in Jesus' image, then setting aside or burying our emotions isn't the path forward. To mature in the image of Christ includes maturing in our emotions. We won't grow out of our emotions. We'll grow out of the immature understanding and expression of our emotions. As we mature, our hearts will begin to beat with passion as God's heart does.

We will, in time, talk about how we can use this amazing gift to have a more truthful understanding of ourselves and our world, but first, we turn to how emotions work and what exactly they communicate.

QUESTIONS FOR REFLECTION

1. Do you find it uncomfortable to consider God as having a full, rich emotional life that spans everything from compassion to hatred? Why, or why not?

2. If you had to choose between a God who is "impassible" (unaffected by emotion and unmoved by us) and a God whom we and our circumstances can move, which would you pick? Why does your choice seem better to you? If you're willing to push deeper, consider what this choice may say about you and your heart.

3. Consider the idea presented in this chapter that God is *omnimotive*, able to contain and feel all emotions without the divine character being compromised or undone. Does this align with what you read in Scripture? How could this idea change your perspective of God and your spiritual life?

Part Three

THE TRUTH IN
YOUR EMOTIONS

Chapter 8

REASON'S SECRET AND EMOTION'S PURPOSE

We are desire. It is the essence of the human soul.…
Absolutely nothing of human greatness is ever accomplished
without it. Not a symphony has been written, a mountain
climbed, an injustice fought, or a love sustained apart from
desire. Desire fuels our search for the life we prize.

John Eldredge, *The Journey of Desire*

I have sought You with all my heart.

Psalm 119:10

Reason has a secret. The key to unlocking it was discovered in the brain of a man named Elliot. Elliot was having headaches. These weren't from stress or a long day staring at a computer screen. The pounding in Elliot's head was so painful, he couldn't function, and it kept getting worse. He finally made a trip to the doctor, and the tests came back with the worst news: Elliot had a brain tumor. The doctors quickly scheduled surgery and successfully removed the tumor.

At first all seemed normal. Elliot was funny and smart, just like before the surgery. As he slowly made his way back into his daily routine, however, something was different. Elliot couldn't seem to organize his life as he did before. He got bogged down in simple decisions. His wife had to remind him to get ready for work. He'd get stuck for hours weighing the pros and cons of trivial decisions like how to sort his files.

It wasn't long before Elliot was let go from his job, and he couldn't hold down any job after that. He entrusted his money to someone untrustworthy. He couldn't follow through on relational commitments. The effort required to get him through the day was overwhelming. In a few years, he had lost his marriage, his life savings, and even a second marriage. He fell off the deep end.

What caused this chain of events? Everyone was stumped. Elliot seemed intelligent and capable. He could talk through the potential consequences of his choices. There didn't seem to be anything wrong with him, yet his daily life was a disaster.

Finally he ended up in the office of Dr. Antonio Damasio, a neurologist and neuroscientist at the University of Iowa. (Dr. Damasio is now the head of the Brain and Creativity Institute at the University of Southern California.) Dr. Damasio and his research team tested Elliot in a hundred ways, trying to figure out what was wrong. Tests showed a high IQ and strong memory and logic. It seemed as though neither the tumor nor the operation had damaged his brain function at all.

Then a member of Dr. Damasio's team suggested one faculty that hadn't been evaluated: Elliot's emotional response. With this evaluation, something strange emerged. Elliot could tell his own tragic life story in detail, but without a hint of anguish, concern, or sadness. No wavering voice, no increased heart rate, no increase in perspiration. None of the normal markers of emotion were present.

Elliot's capacity to feel emotion was just gone. He could explain what good choices looked like, but he had no feeling one way or the other about those choices. He couldn't prioritize between right and wrong or between short-term and long-term gain. The various options of any decision carried no specific emotional significance for him. The surprising result? This deficit left Elliot unable to choose.[1]

REASON'S SECRET

Earlier we discussed how Platonic dualism infected Christian theology, dividing human nature into separate competing parts. This same dualism made its way into other disciplines, including psychology and sociology. A parade of theories have suggested that our minds are split into two parts: creative and linear, emotional and rational, left brained and right brained.[2] But these are just scientific-sounding retreads on the old flesh-and-spirit dualism we inherited from Greek philosophy.

At different times in history, the church ascribed emotions to demons, passions of the flesh, lack of faith, or spiritual immaturity. Similarly, scientists of different eras attributed emotions to an excess of humor, hysterics, out-of-balance brain chemicals, or the residual effect of our evolutionary past. For years researchers said emotions simply couldn't be studied.

What Dr. Damasio discovered with Elliot and other patients with similar brain injuries suggests something else entirely. This new research shows our various mental faculties are woven together into a single integrated whole. Emotions are a type of thought. All thought depends on a more integrated system than we once believed. Our brains have the ability to collect and sort incoming sensory information, weigh its importance, and make decisions based on that analysis. We've always referred to this process as reason. We're only just learning our assumptions were incomplete.

Elliot lost his emotional capacity. The commonly held view suggested this would make him more focused in his decision making, more *reasonable*. After all, emotion could no longer clutter his thinking. The opposite happened. Observing Elliot, Dr. Damasio learned reason's long-kept secret: without emotion, reason is crippled.[3]

As a young man, I idolized Mr. Spock, the pointy-eared first officer from the original *Star Trek* series. As a Vulcan, he was eminently rational, able to see right through the mists of emotion that so often distracted Captain Kirk. Spock's ability seemed like a superpower to me. He was able to cut right to the truth. At the same time, though, Spock was an alien. He didn't understand the emotions of his crew. I felt that way too—like an outsider, not always able to read the emotional tone of a conversation, uncertain of the relational dynamics at play in a group. On the deck of the USS *Enterprise*, Captain Kirk brought passion and intuition. Spock provided careful analysis and logic. When the ship faced a dire crisis, it took Kirk and Spock working together to save the day.

Dr. Damasio and other researchers are showing us this is how our minds work too. While we each have different tendencies and strengths, our ability to make good decisions is the fruit of reason and emotion working together.

When I learned this, it was like finding a missing puzzle piece. I've had a long track record of making emotionally tone-deaf decisions.

I could explain why a certain decision was right. I could marshal the evidence, presenting a solid, often-convincing argument. However, my decisions tended to overlook some vital relational or intuitive element. Decisions that looked so good on paper frequently ended up wrong or, worse, harmful to others. Why had the data failed me? How could I have missed it? Living disconnected from my emotions handicapped my ability to make good decisions.

OUR EMOTIONS ARE PURPOSEFUL

The Genesis creation story tells us God made humans as whole beings, not a composite of separate battling parts. Reason and emotion work hand in hand to provide us with a truthful analysis of what is going on around and within us.

If emotions were created as a part of our nature, they're purposeful. This is true regardless of our beliefs about the origin of humanity. If humanity evolved, then emotions emerged through natural selection because they're crucial for survival. If we were created, then emotions are an integral part of the design our Creator gave us. Either way, emotions are vital for a life well lived.

So what is the purpose of emotions? In this chapter and the next, I'll suggest two. First, emotions move us to act. Why are parents and pastors so concerned about emotional decision making? Because they see emotion often leading young people into destructive choices. They have an emotional reaction. It moves them. Then they act. This is exactly where concerned folks speak up and say, "Well, there's the problem! That's why emotional decisions are bad. Decisions need to be rational, not emotional." We're uncomfortable with our emotions because emotions move us, but this is exactly what they're meant to do.

The word *emotion* derives from the Latin *emovere*, which signifies motion and means "to agitate" or literally "to move out."[4] Emotion is the engine. We can believe and know all sorts of things, but emotion is what moves us to act on what we believe and know. Our emotional responses impart value to the many options we have in any decision. This is the problem Elliot faced. He understood his options. Reason was flooding his mind with data, but without emotion, he became value blind. There was no motivational force empowering him to finally act.

Emotions can surely lead to terrible decisions, but doesn't that just make the point? Emotions motivate us to act, to change things, to finally draw the line at the bottom of our list of pros and cons and get on with living. There's reason to fear that emotion can lead us to destructive ends, but that misses half the story. Emotions can also lead to good decisions, even heroic or godly decisions.

MOVED TOWARD THE GOOD?

In Romans 6, Paul gave a lengthy explanation about how we can avoid sin in our lives. At one point he said this: "Thank God that, although you used to be slaves of sin, you obeyed from the heart that pattern of teaching you were transferred to, and having been liberated from sin, you became enslaved to righteousness."[5]

Paul said we move from being "slaves of sin" to being "enslaved to righteousness." This happens when we obey from the heart. The Greek word for "heart," *kardia,* describes the center of our will as well as our passion and motivation. The obedience Paul spoke of doesn't simply arise from a sense of duty or obligation. Obeying from the heart is when my heart aligns with God's heart. I'm not obeying because a certain behavior is on my church's Good Behavior List. I'm not obeying because I need to prove my value to God or my mom or my pastor. I'm obeying because my heart wants to obey. My feelings are in line with God's feelings.

Parents understand this intuitively. Getting your children to obey you is trivial when you want them to do something they already want to do. Lucas will obey me every time I ask him to eat chocolate. Emerson will obey without question when I ask her to be in charge of something. There's no resistance or talk-back, and the response is immediate. Why? Because my kids' hearts and mine are aligned. One of my goals as a parent is to help my children come to want the things that are good and life giving. Spiritual growth is much the same, the long process of coming to love and desire the things God loves. The more our hearts are aligned with God's, the more our emotions will be like God's. Then obeying God isn't a chore or obligation; it's simply living out what gives us joy.

Hebrews 11 lists many well-known biblical heroes—Enoch, Noah, Abraham, Moses, and others like them. These people were affirmed for their faith, for obeying God in the face of serious obstacles. Verses 15 and 16 say something interesting about how they could move forward with such faith: "If they were thinking about where they came from, they would have had an opportunity to return. But they now desire a better place—a heavenly one."

This is how we move from where we are to where God wants us to be. The first part of the verse speaks to the status quo, life as usual. If these heroes of faith had been thinking about those things, they would have returned to the status quo. Instead of stepping into risk and obedience, they would have gone back to what was comfortable.

But what were they doing? They were longing for "a better place—a heavenly one." This "better place" is where God's will reigns. Jesus called it the "kingdom of God."[6] This new kingdom is where life is lived in alignment with God's heart. These heroes from Scripture weren't just thinking intellectually about that possibility. They were longing, yearning for it. That's emotional desire. You want something so strongly, you stretch yourself in its direction to take hold of it. An emotional response, a yearning for the things of God, drove these people forward.

Matthew Elliott wrote, "Emotions were given to us by God to drive us to our best."[7] The more we feel the way God does, the more our emotions guide us well. Doing Christian life without emotion, or with suppressed emotion, leads us to a drab, brittle life of duty and obligation. When we live cut off from our emotions, we lose the engine intended to drive us Godward. If we try to obey God at all, we trade out passion for duty. That's exactly where I found myself.

THE GARDEN OF GREAT ... JOY?

A dry, legalistic life of obligation is what so many people think Christianity offers, yet that isn't what we see in Scripture at all. Passion lies at the heart of a God-oriented life.

This can be seen even in moments of profound obedience. Think about just one example: Jesus' final, significant decision in the garden of Gethsemane. Soldiers were already on the way to arrest Him. Within hours He would be tortured and then crucified. The Gospels portray Jesus in this moment, not aloof and serene or acting in cold duty. Just the opposite. Jesus was racked with emotional pain and anguish.[8] He didn't want to be alone. He sweat blood.

In the middle of this agony, we get to overhear His prayer: "My Father! If it is possible, let this cup pass from Me." It sounds for all the world like a near emotional breakdown. He was asking to escape the horrors ahead. Was that fear? But then His tone shifted. Jesus decided, "Yet not as I will, but as You will."[9] He submitted to His arrest and the suffering that would follow.

Growing up, I was taught this was an example where Jesus, at the point of greatest temptation, chose to do the right thing. He did His duty. When we look to the text, however, we find something else. The author of Hebrews reflected on Jesus' motivation: "Who for the joy that lay before Him endured a cross and despised the shame and has sat down at the right hand of God's throne."[10]

Wait, what? Why did He do what He did? "For the joy that lay before Him." Did Jesus do the right thing? Yes. Did He do His duty? Yes. But He also did it *for the joy.*

Don't let any theologian tell you differently; joy is an emotion. Jesus had an emotional response to His mission. His heart was moved when He considered God's lost and hurting children, restoring them, bringing healing, and establishing an eternal, new kind of kingdom. In the moment of temptation, Jesus made the right choice, but not only because it was the right choice. Jesus' heart was drawn to the joyful outcome. He was moved.

THE MISSING LINK FOR THE CHURCH

In 2012 I attended the Justice Conference when it was held here in Portland. More than three thousand Christians, including hundreds of pastors, gathered to listen to speakers and discuss how the church could better advocate for justice in our cities. Topics like racism, poverty, homelessness, and mental illness were on the agenda. The room hummed with the vibrant energy of people longing to change the world.

In conversations between sessions and over meals, a theme emerged. The people at this conference were already convinced, excited to move forward. They were also frustrated, even sad, because folks in their home congregations didn't have the same energy, commitment, or understanding. Over and over I heard the same complaint: How is it possible the Bible is so clear about our calling to justice yet the Christians in our churches just aren't interested?

I had a moment of déjà vu on the drive home. I remembered being a young pastor attending church-leadership conferences almost two decades earlier. In similar halls, thousands of pastors gathered to listen to speakers and discuss how the church could be better at evangelism. But over lunch and in the conversations between sessions, I heard the same complaint: How is it possible the Bible is so clear about our calling to evangelize the world yet most Christians just aren't interested?

Those church-growth conferences and the Justice Conference were on different ends of the church-world spectrum. The kinds of people present and the churches they represented were in some ways worlds apart. Yet the same question emerged. How is it this cause is so vital, so clearly biblical, yet people just don't seem interested? Both groups had the same problem. The problem wasn't a lack of scriptural support or clear teaching. The problem wasn't about *reasons* at all. The problem was emotional.

Most of us simply don't feel as God does about these matters. If your church's first priority is evangelism but you don't feel moved on behalf of people who don't know Christ, then you won't evangelize. You may do it for a time, out of obligation or duty, but you won't last. You'll decide you don't have the gift. You'll justify yourself, saying the best evangelism is just being kind. No amount of biblical teaching will change the situation, because the problem isn't in your head. It's in your heart. You don't feel as God does.

If your church's priority is justice, the same problem exists. Learn the facts about racism or homelessness or poverty. Memorize scriptures about standing up for the widow and orphan. It won't make a difference. Until your heart is moved for people in the margins, you won't act.

Liberal, conservative, or in between, congregations are facing the same problem. It's a problem of the heart. Because emotion has been left out of the conversation of discipleship, most of us don't feel as God does. Without this emotional connection, we simply aren't moved to act.

PUSHED ACROSS THE LINE

As I look back at some of the turning-point decisions in my life, I'm humbled. I've lived most of my life hypercontrolled, with emotions untrusted and deeply buried. I thought I was making carefully considered decisions based on thorough analysis, but in truth, emotions have been a deep part of all my decisions. Turns out, the prejudice I've carried against emotions all these years is irrational. The painful irony!

Why did I leave architecture school, a long-term plan I worked hard to achieve, to go into the ministry? Because I was compelled.

Why did I leave the denomination of my family and childhood, a community where I had a clear career path, to join a nondenominational church plant with no job security? Because of longing.

Why did my wife and I choose to spend a small fortune to adopt our son, Lucas? Because I was so profoundly grateful for the family who took the same risk with me.

Why did I become the de facto parent for a homeless teenager, inviting all his chaos into my life? Because of compassion. My heart ached for his pain, and I longed for him to know love.

Why do I continue in the crazy job of pastoring, with long hours and overwhelming expectations? Because I long for that same better place from Hebrews 11, where people find wholeness and passion, living out God's heart in this world.

I came to see that the very best choices I've ever made—the moments when perhaps my heart was aligned most with God's—all grew out of passion or desire. Did I have rational explanations and justifications for those choices? Of course! I had lists, charts, and reasons. Did I have Scripture I could cite? Yep. Was there a sense of the Holy Spirit's leading? Sometimes. But what always drew me to cross the line was an emotion that carried me into obedience or nudged me to take a risk. Upon reflection, you might see this is true of your life as well.

We're faced with choices every day. Each choice can be a step toward numbness and dryness until all we're left with is duty. Take that path, and you'll miss God's best for you.

How is it some followers of Jesus choose to travel across the world, facing deprivation and danger to share the gospel? How is it there are people who give their lives and resources to serve the poor, the sick, or those in prison? How is it there are teachers who choose to work for unfair wages to give children a better future? How is it some people stand up to power, risking their lives and positions to speak out for those who have no voice?

Maybe those examples seem too big for you, so start smaller. How is it some give sacrificially, or even just tithe their income when things are tight? How is it others stick with a wounded marriage that has a long path toward healing? How is it people go through the painful conversations needed for reconciliation?

It doesn't happen because of duty, at least not over time. You won't be a lasting influence for good in this world, in your neighborhood, or even in your family because of obligation. You won't take the kinds of risks that lead to growth and transformation just because it's the right thing to do. Every great deed ever done for God grew from passion. The act was motivated by an emotional response—shaped by Scripture, informed by God's character, held accountable by truth, but an emotional response nonetheless. A faithful life starts with a heart beating in rhythm with God's heart, becoming passionate about what God is passionate about.

This is why the conversation about emotion matters. This is why growing emotionally is part of discipleship. This is why it's so vital for followers of Jesus to find healing for our emotional and relational brokenness. This is why churches must set aside expectations of perfection and allow people to be real about their weakness and fear.

The old myth is half right. Emotions do lead us. They can certainly lead us to pain or destruction, but they can just as well lead us into greatness, faithfulness, mercy, and grace. That is their purpose.

QUESTIONS FOR REFLECTION

1. The first purpose of emotion is to move us. How have you seen this play out in your life? When has emotion moved you in a negative or destructive direction? When has it moved you in a positive, life-giving, or God-honoring direction?

2. We tend to act based on three motivations: duty (doing something because it's the right thing), obligation (doing something because of a stated or unstated commitment), or desire (doing something because we want to). Think of examples in your life when you acted from each of these motivations. How were those experiences different?

3. Imagine you woke up one morning and a miracle had happened overnight. Your heart had changed. Suddenly you find that you naturally and authentically love the things God loves. How do you imagine your life would be different? What would godly obedience feel like?

Chapter 9

YOUR EMOTIONS ALWAYS TELL YOU THE TRUTH ...

We listen for guidance everywhere except from within.
Parker J. Palmer, *Let Your Life Speak*

Who put wisdom in the heart?
Job 38:36

I told you emotions serve two purposes in our lives. The first we talked about in the last chapter: emotions exist to move us. The second purpose, though, is a much harder sell.

Elizabeth Johnston and Leah Olson, in their insightful book *The Feeling Brain*, summarize the complex emotional-response system this way: "Organisms are continually bombarded by a wealth of information—from outside and inside the body and brain—and emotions provide a way of evaluating and prioritizing what to respond to."[1] Simply put, our emotions exist to tell us the truth. In fact, our emotions always tell us the truth.

When I say this, I invariably get a reaction. How can emotions tell the truth? Aren't they subjective? What about fallen human nature? We've all experienced situations where our emotions clouded the truth. Common sense tells us we can't let emotions clutter our decision making. Telling people to just follow their feelings sounds like such terrible advice—and it is.

The problem isn't with emotions, however. As we unpack the inner workings of our emotional-response system, you will see that it is designed to give us feedback on our external circumstances and our internal states. Disruptions like trauma, substance abuse, and mental illness can certainly compromise this system. For most of us, the vast majority of the time, however, this feedback is truthful, but there's a catch. *It's just not always the truth we think.* Sometimes we hear wrong. Sometimes we misunderstand. Sometimes our emotions are telling us something we didn't expect or don't want to face.

Think back to the aftermath of my meeting with the church board members when I felt so desperate. I was sitting in my car, holding on to the steering wheel for dear life, trying to force back the angry tears. My body was responding to my circumstances. My gut was tight. Nausea crept in. I had a lump in my throat and heavy pressure on my shoulders. Heat radiated through my neck into my face, a warning of the tears that were moments away.

My mind was responding too. A high-speed kaleidoscope of thoughts and mental images overwhelmed me: Feelings of failure. Fear of what Christina would say when I told her. Frustration that I didn't feel heard. Self-recrimination growling, *I should never have said anything*. A growing sense of resolve to just work harder. A competing sense of desperation. I was already working as hard as I could! Then hopelessness. The processes unfolding in my body and mind were the manifestation of emotion, but I wasn't practiced in listening to or understanding those signs. To me, it was all just discomfort, conflict, and pressure.

The emotional energy of fear, sadness, and anger was pushing me toward action. I wanted to drive home and write a blazing letter of resignation. I had served these people for more than a decade. I'd walked with them through crisis and trauma. I'd answered late-night calls and met with them when it fit their schedules, at the expense of my own family. But when my life was coming off the rails, I was just supposed to work harder, prioritize better, and attend fewer meetings? I wanted to tell them exactly where they could go!

My emotions were moving me to act. At the same time, they were also telling me the truth. But I was broken and inexperienced at listening to my emotions. As I've said, the truth our emotions carry isn't always the truth we think, nor is it often the truth we want to hear.

TIME TO CHECK YOUR ENGINE

Every car has one enigmatic warning light on the dashboard: the check-engine light. Think about how you relate to it. Our parents and unread car manuals told us that when this light comes on, we need to pull over immediately. We're putting our car in dire risk if we keep driving. Who knows? The engine might be moments away from blowing up. Most of the time nothing disastrous happens—at least not immediately. With no clear consequence, the check-engine light loses its motivational power. Maybe it's important, but we're on our way somewhere. We'll deal with it next week.

What do you do when the check-engine light comes on? Do you drive your car straight to the shop? Or do you shift into hope and denial? Maybe when you start your car tomorrow, the light won't be glowing.

Instead of seeing the check-engine light as a helpful warning, many of us experience it as an irritant. It likely means a trip to the mechanic we don't have time or money for. So when that light comes on, some of us just cross our fingers. Delusion isn't a helpful strategy for car maintenance or for mental health. The check-engine light always tells us the truth. But most of the time, we don't know what that truth is.

There's a way to find out. The repair shop (or your mechanic neighbor, if you're lucky) has a little device that plugs into your car's onboard computer. Within a few seconds, the device flashes a special code. Maybe a valve is sticking, or there's a vacuum leak. I have a friend whose car triggers the check-engine light when the gas cap isn't on tight enough. Each of these might not be a crisis, but left unattended, some of these seemingly small issues can lead to danger.

ALWAYS TRUE, BUT NOT ALWAYS CLEAR

Sitting in that car after my meeting, all my personal check-engine lights were on: the tightness in my chest, the sick feeling in my stomach, the lump in my throat, the feeling of pressure on my shoulders, the tears. My body was showing the physical indicators of stress and fear. My mind was racing, trying to provide me with an explanation and a course of action. Everything happening to me just then was normal.

Our brains and bodies are programmed to seek survival. Discomfort means something appears to be threatening our optimum survival. For example, if the discomfort is external, like the freezing cold of winter, your brain and body initiate a survival sequence. First, you experience peripheral vasoconstriction. The blood vessels in your limbs begin to tighten, limiting the flow of blood to your extremities. This keeps the warm blood in your core, where it's needed to protect your vital organs. Then you begin to shiver, which produces heat. At the same time, you become aware that you're cold and need to find shelter.

If the discomfort is internal, like fear, your brain and body go through a similar sequence. Your vision focuses. Blood flows away from your stomach toward the large muscles in your legs and arms. Adrenaline is released into your bloodstream, causing your heart to beat harder and faster. Your blood-sugar level jumps, providing an immediate boost of energy. As the physiological fight-or-flight response kicks in, you become aware of danger and immediately begin to desire safety.

In any situation of discomfort, your brain and body start triggering check-engine lights all over the place. Pay attention. Do something! Sometimes the solution is obvious. If it's freezing, get a jacket. Go inside. Start a fire. When the check-engine light is lit up because of emotional discomfort, interpreting the meaning is much more complex.

In my car after that board meeting, I experienced emotional stress. I was angry I hadn't been heard. I was anxious this meeting meant I'd have to work harder, which I already knew I couldn't do. I was terrified of failure, afraid I'd crash in some horrible way, hurting my family or the church. But in the moment, I wasn't conscious of any of this. I was frustrated, feeling alone and hopeless.

My emotional-response system had initiated the fight-or-flight protocol. Instead of being able to think through the situation clearly, I had mental tunnel vision. Instead of being compassionately aware of the board members' perspectives, I was blinded by my own need for relief. I felt urgency as I drove away from that meeting.

My emotions were moving me toward action: quit, blame others for my situation, make a series of furious phone calls. Each of these options was a way to sidestep or displace my own discomfort as quickly as I could. My emotions were also giving me truth. Something in my circumstances needed to change, and desperately. But if I had acted on what first came to mind, I would have made a terrible mistake. My immediate interpretation of the truth wasn't accurate.

UNDERSTANDING THE WARNING LIGHT

To get ahold of the truth our emotions are telling us, we have to understand them a bit better—how they work, where they come from, and what they mean.

The fact is that few of us have ever been taught about our emotions. We have years of schooling that teach us how to reason. In the church, we provide sermons, classes, and programs so people can learn how to follow Jesus. You can hire a nutritionist to teach you how to feed your body and a personal trainer to teach you how to be fit. When it comes to emotions, we think we understand them because they're so intense and personal—but the evidence of our choices says something different.

If we want to understand the warning lights on our cars' dashboards, we need to learn more about what goes on under the hood. Emotions are the same. We don't need to be afraid or confused when our emotional check-engine lights come on. When we understand something of how our emotions work and why, we can begin to understand the truth they're delivering to us.

IS THIS EXPERIENCE GOOD FOR ME OR BAD FOR ME?

All emotions start with a push or a pull. When I say emotions exist to move us, this push or pull is what gets the movement rolling. Fear, disgust, and shame push us away from certain things. Intrigue, joy, and love pull us toward other things.[2] Our bodies and minds are wired to seek well-being. This balanced state, as well as the internal mechanisms and drives regulating the process, is referred to as homeostasis. When everything works as it should, we're drawn toward what provides for the best quality of life and repulsed by what could endanger us.

Our emotional responses are part of this system. At the simplest level, we have emotional responses to our immediate circumstances and internal states. Is this change in circumstance or internal state good or bad for us? If it's good and supportive, healthy emotions should draw us toward the new stimulus with affection, happiness, satisfaction, or joy. If the change is dangerous or threatening, our emotions are meant to repel us from the stimulus with responses like anxiety, fear, disgust, and hate.

If an emotional response is confusing or overwhelming, two simple questions will help to bring clarity:

1. Am I feeling pulled toward something or pushed away from something?
2. What is the object I'm reacting to? Why?

If you're feeling torn or trapped, unable to make a decision, it's possible you're simultaneously experiencing an emotional pull toward one aspect of your situation and a competing push away from something else. Being able to identify where and why you feel pulled or pushed can clear away much of your mental fog.

These questions also point out something vital. Your emotions are not you. Your feelings are information, a kind of knowledge. They aren't bad or shameful. They're a check-engine light inviting your attention. Knowing this dramatically lowered my anxiety about emotions, enabling me to begin thinking about what I was feeling rather than being driven into a reaction.

Grasping this push-pull dynamic is the first building block in understanding what our emotions are telling us, but there is so much more. Next, let's lift up the hood and take a look at the inner workings of our emotional-response system.

QUESTIONS FOR REFLECTION

1. What was your reaction when you read that your emotions always tell you the truth? Why did you have this response? Many people have a strong negative reaction. Of course, the sentence is intentionally provocative. The goal is to cause you to reflect on your own predisposition about emotions. Having heard more about how emotions function in the body and the brain, how does this alter your predisposition?

2. The first principle to understand about emotions is that all emotions are either a push away from something or a pull toward something. How might knowing this change the way you relate to your emotions?

3. Emotions are information. They provide feedback about your internal state and external circumstances. How does knowing this change the way you see your own emotions? Someone else's?

Chapter 10

SEEING THE INNER WORKINGS

The heart has its reasons, which reason does not know.

Blaise Pascal, *Pensées*

Keep your heart with all vigilance, for from it flow the springs of life.

Proverbs 4:23 NRSV

What actually happens when we feel an emotion? There are many theories about this. For most of human history, the internal mechanisms of emotion have been invisible, but in recent years, dramatic innovations in brain research have given neuroscientists the ability to test their theories.

The current best hypothesis about the inner workings of emotions goes like this: Emotions are composite experiences. Each emotion, like joy or fear, is a nearly simultaneous cluster of body postures, brain chemicals, neurological signals, sensations, and thoughts forming a recognizable pattern. When a healthy person encounters a stimulus, these responses are predictable. Some of these patterns

seem hardwired into us. Others are learned through repeated expo-
sure. These response patterns rapidly induce a change of state in our
bodies and minds. This change of state is how we become aware we
are feeling an emotion.[1]

Emotions include a collection of responses happening in the
body. The brain releases certain chemicals. Specific neurons fire.
Particular physiological responses, like muscle contractions, take
place. The body takes on a recognizable stance.

These physical states seem to be nearly universal among humans
and are common even with some animals. Lips pull back from the
teeth in rage. Eyes open wide in a moment of surprise. We've seen
these responses in our pets, in gorillas, even in our two-year-old children. When we see their bodies take on these familiar postures, we
immediately know something about what they're experiencing.

A collection of thoughts emerge in connection with these body
states—dark and heavy thoughts or excited and uplifting thoughts.
These thoughts come into being almost simultaneously with the
changes in our bodies.[2] The relationship between body state and
internal feeling is fantastically interesting. The insight we now have,
thanks to the innovations of brain imagery, tells us these two aspects
of our emotional-response system are inextricably linked, and in
some unexpected ways.

I enjoyed the detective show *Lie to Me*.[3] The protagonist, Dr. Cal
Lightman, was an expert in microexpressions, the tiny unconscious
ways emotion shows up in our bodies. This knowledge let him get
inside criminals' minds, cracking open his cases. Turns out, his
character was loosely based on a real researcher, Dr. Paul Ekman. In
multiple studies, Ekman demonstrated something unexpected: we

experience emotions in our bodies before we are consciously aware of them. Sounds backward, but it's true.

In one study Ekman asked participants to arrange their facial muscles in a certain manner. They were given mechanical instructions to move the muscles in their faces, such as "Pull your eyebrows down and together. Narrow your lips and press them together." No instructions about emotions were given. Emotions weren't even mentioned. Yet when the subjects were asked about their emotional states following the exercise, 78 percent reported feeling the expected emotion for the facial expression they had been guided to form.[4] The body posture not only preceded the conscious experience of emotion but actually evoked it.[5]

Another research team showed subjects photos of faces. Most of the photos showed faces with a neutral expression, but interspersed were photos of ecstatic or terrified faces. These emotionally evocative pictures were shown so quickly that most subjects reported never seeing them. Yet functional magnetic resonance imaging (fMRI) scans showed the amygdala was more active when the fearful images were shown. This was true even for subjects who had no conscious awareness of having seen anything other than the emotionally neutral faces.[6] Their bodies were showing awareness of an emotional threat that their conscious minds had not yet identified! Our emotions aren't just subjective mental experiences—all in the mind—but are connected deeply to our bodies and our physical sense of the circumstances we find ourselves in.

Our conscious experience of emotion is the proverbial tip of the iceberg. Studies like these hint at the inner workings of emotion and intuition. In fact, intuition isn't some magical ability given to special people. This is something God built into each of us, something we can learn to listen to. That's wonderful news, especially for someone as emotionally immature and unpracticed as I was.

THE SEQUENCE OF YOUR EMOTIONAL-RESPONSE SYSTEM

Our ability to listen well to this guidance and use it constructively begins with keeping in mind the sequence of the emotional-response system. Every emotional experience can be understood as a composite of four separate but connected events:

1. We experience a change of body state.
2. We experience a collection of thoughts.
3. Those thoughts focus on an object.
4. We generate a story about what just happened.

In our conscious experience, these events seem to happen simultaneously. They generally proceed in this order, even if they're separated only by nearly imperceptible gaps. Let me walk you through how this sequence unfolded for me recently.

First comes the change in body state. This morning I read an email on my phone. As I read, my gut tensed. The message was a sharp rebuke from a coworker who was hurt and angry. While reading the accusatory words, I noticed a heaviness settle in my chest, and my shoulders tightened. These are my first signs of anxiety.[7] I knew a complicated, probably painful conversation was coming. I had said something that unintentionally created fear and anger for someone I care about. It was a miscommunication, but it was also clearly my fault.

Second, a collection of thoughts emerges, mirroring the body state and ushering in a certain tone of mind. As I anticipated the conflict scenario, my thoughts grew anxious. *Ugh. This is not going to be fun. I wonder if this is what gets me fired. Maybe we won't be friends anymore.* My insecurities charged forward, with my mental space becoming uncertain and agitated.

(Even as I write this description, the same emotions are rising again. The pace and depth of my breathing changed just now, and my stomach has tightened in the last couple of minutes—and all from reflecting on something I experienced several hours ago.)

Third, a stark awareness surfaces of the object we believe triggered our emotional response, and mental tunnel vision kicks in. As anxiety flooded my mind, my thoughts locked on the conversation that created this miscommunication. The person's pinched look of disappointment, projected broadly across the theater of my mind, replayed on a mental loop. More specifically, the object of my emotional response became my coworker's anger and frustration with me.

Finally, we generate a mental narrative, a story explaining why the object caused this response. This story has a plot. Even though it emerges instantly and we can often express it with just a handful of words, there's a whole narrative arc. "He attacked me!" "What a nice surprise! She must like me." These stories feel true, but they may not reflect our real circumstances. This is the part of the sequence when it's best to be circumspect with ourselves. Our brains deeply detest discomfort. In our rush to feel better, we often leap to judgments, and then actions, without considering all the facts.

In the case of my email, the risk for me was blaming my discomfort on the person I had interacted with. Disappointing people is painful for me. Far less painful is blame. Stories emerged rapidly in my mind: *This person has always been too demanding.... He cornered me in an unfair way.... If he had the slightest bit of Christian grace, he wouldn't have misinterpreted my words.* My mind rushed to replace my accurate sense of guilt with a dishonest sense of indignation and blame. (Even as I type, I can feel the energy within me building against that person.) If I didn't take time to interrogate my feelings, I might already have conceded to this interpretation. I would certainly feel better with an invigorating whiff of righteous indignation. Anger is almost always less painful than guilt.

You may notice I haven't included any action or response in this sequence of events. Emotions always move us to act, so why wouldn't the action be included? Simple. Whatever action we choose isn't compulsory. These four linked events are nearly simultaneous and mostly automatic. In most cases, they happen *to* us.[8] They're not a moral choice, not sin. They are sensory responses to our external circumstances and internal states in much the same way a thermometer reads temperature. Even our immediate response of identifying an object of the emotion and creating a story is in some sense automatic. It's possible for us to take control of the process in this later stage, but even so, our minds make the associations they make. Until we've invested time and attention learning how to listen to our emotions, even this part of the process is involuntary and nearly instantaneous.

A clear gap exists between this process and our response. When we act or speak or raise a fist, we're making a conscious choice. The emotion may have moved us, but now we're choosing how we'll spend that emotional energy. We choose, even if the choice feels instant and reactive. In some ways, the path of both emotional maturity and spiritual maturity can be described as a journey to create a thoughtful space between the emotional motivation and the response.

My emotional response to that painful email generated a turbulent pool of energy. Only action could dissipate it. A fast-paced, cut-scene montage of choices flooded my mind: Slam my smartphone on the table in a burst of anger. Call this person and give him an earful for his ungracious assumptions. Write an email to the board explaining my actions, justifying my behavior, and inoculating myself against blame.

None of these options for action were automatic, even though they automatically came to mind. I had the ability to choose. I needed to take responsibility, own how I had created the circumstance, and apologize. Perhaps we could navigate our way through the discomfort to reconciliation. That kind of response isn't automatic for me or for most of us. That's why the action we choose is separate from the sequence of the emotional response.

Just to make sure I'm not creating a false picture of myself, let me say this: I don't always choose such a mature path. Many times, often with those closest to me, my reactions still get the better of me. I often choose the shortsighted, selfish path of defensiveness or anger. Yet the more I've learned about my emotions, the more I know I have the ability to choose how I respond.

DIFFERENT EMOTIONS CARRY DIFFERENT INFORMATION

A change happens in our external circumstances or internal states. Our emotions respond. The sequence unfolds: First, there is a change

in body state. Almost simultaneously, a cocktail of thoughts associated with those bodily responses emerges. Then we become aware of
the object we're reacting to with a gut-level sense of push or pull. This
leads to the near-immediate formulation of a story explaining what
we're feeling and why. All of this is usually experienced in almost
simultaneous succession.

This process can deliver an incredibly wide range of information. We have many different emotions. Those emotions can
have different meanings in different contexts. Sometimes we feel
multiple emotions simultaneously, or even conflicting emotions,
which makes life all the more exciting—or confusing.

Quite a number of researchers and theorists have devised ways
of categorizing emotions. These lists are never entirely accurate or
comprehensive, but they can be helpful as you begin paying attention to your emotions. The framework I found most helpful is called
Plutchik's Wheel of Emotions.[9]

Dr. Robert Plutchik suggested there are eight basic emotions—
terror, rage, vigilance, amazement, ecstacy, grief, admiration, and
loathing—which he presented in four pairs: anger and fear, anticipation and surprise, joy and sadness, trust and disgust (see table 1). You
may even notice the push and pull in each pairing.

Anger and fear are responses to a threat, obstacle, or violation.
One response retreats from the object; the other aggressively moves
toward it. Anticipation and surprise are responses to something
new or uncertain. Anticipation is what we feel as we head into
new territory. Surprise is the response we feel when confronted
with the unexpected. Joy and sadness are responses connected to
what we hold dear. We feel sadness when we lose something that

matters to us; joy emerges when we gain something important. Trust and disgust are emotional responses related to acceptance and connection. Trust is the emotion that draws us toward something or someone we accept and feel connected to. Disgust is the response that pushes us away from something unpalatable or socially unacceptable.

Emotion	Content	How We See the Object	Our Intuitive Response
Emotions are not subjective, but our interpretations are. Remember that we define our emotions always in relationship to our own view of the circumstances. A good way to keep this in mind is to describe each emotion with the sentence "_____ is the emotion you feel when, in your own personal logic, you or someone or something that matters to you has been _____."			
anger	violated or obstructed	enemy	fight (pull toward)
fear	threatened	danger	flight (push away)
anticipation	exploring new terrain	intriguing	explore (pull toward)
surprise	encountering the unexpected	unexpected	stop to check (push away)
joy	experiencing gain	possessed	exclaim, repeat behavior (pull toward)
sadness	experiencing loss	beyond reach	cry, shut down (push away)
trust	experiencing acceptance and inclusion	friend	nurture (pull toward)
disgust	contaminated	unacceptable	reject, exclude (push away)

Adapted from Plutchik's Eight Primary Emotions
Table 1

These eight emotions behave like the primary colors. When these emotions combine, they provide the rich palette of emotional responses

we all experience. Plutchik created a three-dimensional diagram showing how emotions can blend and change with varying degrees of
intensity (see figure 1).[10]

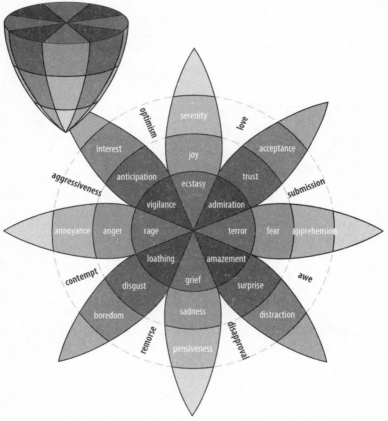

Figure 1: Plutchik's Wheel of Emotions[11]

The eight core emotions are found in the first ring. Extending the
circle as a three-dimensional cone accounts for intensity. The emotions in the center are the most intense, and they decrease in intensity
as the cone narrows. For example, annoyance is the emotion of anger

at lowest intensity, while rage is anger at full bore. Sadness can be experienced as low-intensity pensiveness or high-intensity grief.

The model also shows how the primary emotions combine to create more complex emotions. Surprise blended with fear gives us awe or alarm. Anger mixed with disgust yields the relationally devastating emotion of contempt. Interestingly, Plutchik suggested that love is the blending of trust and joy—feeling both acceptance and the fullness of having what you desire.

Of course, emotional categorizations like this aren't a science. They're more like high-level maps helping us get into the right neighborhood. For those of us who have spent a lifetime numb to the rich meaning of our emotions, tools like this can be helpful maps for navigating unfamiliar territory.

SO WHERE IS THE TRUTH?

I said earlier that our emotions always tell the truth. Given the sequence of events that make up our emotional responses and the inevitable subjectivity in interpreting this information, how can this possibly be the case?

There are undoubtedly times when our emotional-response systems are compromised. We're not perfect. Trauma, substance abuse, mental illness, distraction, and even stress can alter the way we experience and understand our emotions. In these cases, the truth our emotions carry can get twisted. Also, our capacity to interpret emotions is cumulatively built by our life experience. Years of badly interpreted emotions can make it difficult to see our own emotions clearly.

Even so, for most of us, this sequence of events is predictable and carries important information about our lives and circumstances. Like the warning light on the dash of our cars, it always tells us something true. Something has occurred in our hearts or circumstances. We may not correctly understand what our emotions convey, but they point toward something needing our attention.

The anxiety that surfaced when I read that email was truthful information. Anxiety is a low-grade form of fear. I was experiencing a threat. I could have blamed the person for my discomfort, but as I sat with the emotion—a process that included reflection, journaling, and prayer—I was able to hear truth. My own choices hurt someone I cared about. It was a miscommunication, but it had real relational consequences. Seeing those consequences and the role I played threatened my sense of security. Anxiety pointed me toward a deeper fear—the fear of being unmasked, exposed, and excluded. The circumstance wasn't likely to cause this sort of outcome, but this fear is embedded deeply in my personal story, a hot button in me that's easy to push. Then I often overreact in an effort to reestablish a sense of security.

My initial emotional response truthfully indicated that something critical had happened in my relational life. Anxiety indicated I was feeling threatened. My emotions pointed to this person as the object, more specifically to his disappointment in me. This was truthful in the immediate sense. I had disappointed him. It was also truthful in a deeper, more important sense. Disappointing people is painful for me. My emotional response was a truthful flag marking an unhealed wound from my personal story. Even the energy this emotional response evoked, the energy that moved me to act, was right. I needed to do something about this! I was being moved to seek forgiveness and reconciliation. God was using an emotional experience and my reflection on it to correct and grow me.

Understanding the sequence of our emotional-response system provides questions that can help us understand our emotions better and discern truth within them.

- **My body is responding in a certain way. Why is this happening at this particular moment?** For example: tightened chest, sense of heaviness in my gut, labored breathing, feeling of weight on my shoulders, etc. What do these physiological responses indicate?

- **My thoughts are showing up in a certain way. Why is this happening just now?** For example: I'm having thoughts that are fretful, defensive, anxious, blaming. Or my thoughts are filled with anticipation, excitement, or happiness. What do these thoughts indicate?

- **A particular object (person, event, experience) is occupying my thoughts. Why is this happening at this particular moment? Am I feeling some kind of push away from or pull toward this object?** For example: *I need to get away from this person.* Or *I'm feeling like I must stand up and speak.* Or *I want to hold on to this moment.*

- **My story right now is ... Why is this story emerging in my mind just now?** For example: *This person wronged me. This person loves me. This event was unfair. This option is right for me.*

WHY WE CAN NEVER JUST IGNORE OUR EMOTIONS

Perhaps all of this seems like an awful lot of work. If you're not used to doing it, it can be. Shortly after the pastoral retreat in Minnesota, I had a catastrophe of a conversation with someone. (It seems to be a theme in my life, doesn't it? I'm learning that the more out of touch I am with my emotions, the less relationally intuitive I'll be.) But this time I was armed with new tools and information, so I sat down to untangle what had happened and why. I reflected, prayed, and journaled about the conversation, thinking through those questions. When I was finished, I was surprised to see that I not only had a clearheaded understanding of the situation, but I also had landed on a path forward with the person.

This was great news. I'd never had this kind of emotional clarity before. At the same time, though, I was frustrated. The process had taken hours. I didn't have time to journal like this through every emotionally charged incident. I imagined my life grinding to a halt with every conflict as I call for a time-out to go sit with a candle and my journal. I couldn't afford that!

As I applied myself to this process, however, I saw again what we already know. As with any skill, the more we use it, the faster and more intuitive it becomes. It's slow and ungainly at first only because we don't know what we're doing. For some of us, new muscles are getting a workout, but this is a workout worth doing. This isn't just a metaphor. As we use these tools, our brains actually change. New neural pathways come online. With practice, we can find a level of personal insight not available any other way. This process allows us to bring the deepest parts of ourselves before God in a way that can result in real growth.

Frankly, if we aren't willing to tackle the task of growing emotionally, there will be painful consequences in our lives. Emotional immaturity pushes us into poorly lived lives. The instinct to avoid discomfort can drive us toward choices with short-term benefits. These choices are often the most self-indulgent or addictive. Over time they pile up, resulting in fragile, insecure, and inauthentic lives.

It may sound noble to ignore emotions. Trying to live by reason or truth alone seems elevated, more spiritual. But this is just not the case. If someone told you the most spiritual way to move around was to hop on one leg, you would know immediately that this person was off the deep end. Choosing to live without carefully considering our emotional responses is just as absurd. Drivers who ignore the check-engine light on the dash are naive, irresponsible, and even a threat to those around them. Emotions are meant to bring to mind crucial information about our hearts and circumstances. Carefully handled, they are messengers of truth. Giving proper and appropriate attention to our emotions is one of the ways we learn and grow. It's also one of the places the Holy Spirit works most deeply in our lives.

QUESTIONS FOR REFLECTION

1. Emotions are composite experiences that include a change of body state, a set of thoughts, an identified object, and an explanatory story. Have you ever thought about your emotions in this way? How might this framework change the way you relate to emotions?

2. What did you find interesting or helpful in the basic emotions chart or Plutchik's Wheel of Emotions?

3. If God designed our emotions to function in a predictable way, they can be studied and learned from. What might this mean regarding the role of emotions in the process of personal or spiritual growth?

Chapter 11

WHEN YOU'RE CALLED TO FIGHT

A man that does not know how to be angry,
does not know how to be good.

Henry Ward Beecher, "Moth-Eaten Garments"

Be angry and do not sin.

Ephesians 4:26

Deep within your brain lies a paired bundles of cells, roughly the shape of almonds. This tiny brain structure has been a cast member in every drama during your life. This is your amygdala. It's not fair to blame the amygdala for all your difficulties. It's also kept you alive. This is the hair trigger for your fight-or-flight response. Something startling happens. Before your conscious mind has time to sort and interpret what happened, your amygdala has already raised the alarm.[1]

Your body responds to that alarm with urgent action. Hormones are pumped into the bloodstream. Your heartbeat and pace of breathing accelerate. Blood flow is redirected. Energy, in the form of blood sugar, is released to your large muscles. As your body jolts into this posture, your conscious mind becomes aware of potential danger. Only now do your thoughts begin to catch up. This burst of activity and energy, called hyperarousal, means something—but what? That depends entirely on the interpretation extracted from the information pouring into your brain.

Is an enemy attacking? Is something intangible but precious, like your pride, getting beaten up? If your mind's interpretation of the data leans toward danger, then the feeling you experience is fear. An urge to flee will come over you. If the danger has already struck and the interpretation is that you or someone you love has been violated, then the feeling you experience is anger. You'll experience a surge of energy and a desire to fight.

Here we see the link between two of our most powerful emotions, anger and fear. Both responses originate from our perspective that we've been threatened, obstructed, or violated in some way. Fear pushes us away, hopefully toward safety. Anger pulls us forward, intent on stopping the attack.

Because fear and anger both have to do with safety, they have enormous power over us. They are deeply uncomfortable. Most of us are highly motivated to make the sensations stop. This drive can overwhelm our good intentions, veto our sense of right and wrong, even obscure our view of what is safe or healthy in the long term. These two emotions so predictably short-circuit good decision making, they are the easiest paths to manipulating us. Emotions that scare us and create a sense of urgency can get us to do almost anything, even betray our own long-term security. Politicians, con men, even some preachers, are skilled at leveraging these emotions against us.

In spite of the risks, these two emotions are vital. They are God-given gifts meant to tell us something important about ourselves and our environment. Without fear, we couldn't quickly discern danger. Without anger, we would rarely be motivated to stand against injustice.

THE POWER OF ANGER

Anger can be painful, confusing, and scary. It causes conflict and clouds our judgment. It also makes us feel powerful, moves us to action, and ignites a fire that makes change happen.

Every one of us experiences anger, but how we handle it has much to do with our personal stories. Some of us grew up in homes where expressing anger wasn't allowed. We learned to contain it, like holding a beach ball underwater. Others grew up in angry homes, where rage was a form of communication. Anger has become such a part of how we relate to the world, we don't even know we're feeling it. When asked if we're angry, we're surprised by the question, perhaps even offended. For some of us, anger is tied up with abuse. Every time we or someone else gets angry, fear clutches our hearts. For others, anger is a force of passion, a power to be harnessed.

All of us have to figure out what to do with anger in our lives. Is anger a sin? Is it not? Does it serve a purpose in our lives? How can it possibly reflect the image of God?

For a long time, anger was the only high-intensity emotion I could feel. Perhaps it's more accurate to say that all high-intensity emotion felt like anger to me. Something would happen that should have made me sad or afraid. Instead, I just felt angry. Even now, after years of counseling and hard work, I will sometimes find myself angry and have to slowly unpack my thoughts to discover the other emotions waiting to be heard beneath anger's fiery armor.

Anger is simply the feeling you get when you've been violated.*[2] That asterisk adds a crucial clause: "according to your own private logic."[3] Anger emerges when you *perceive* you've been hurt, offended, or violated or when your will has been obstructed. Maybe the offense really happened, or maybe it's just your own perception. Either way, this angry feeling boils up from within.

For years I was an avid paintball player. Paintball is a great illustration of the involuntary nature of anger. On the field, with paintballs flying at you at 275 feet per second, your field of vision narrows. In that hyperfocused state, it's easy to miss an opponent sneaking up on your flank. When that jerk shoots you unexpectedly, it hurts like nothing else! Worse, compounding the hurt is a blast of brain chemicals and an instantaneous emotional reaction. You go from stealthy ninja to raging idiot in a fraction of a second. I've seen players angrily rip off their protective face masks, putting their eyes in danger, or slam paint markers worth hundreds of dollars into the nearest tree while screaming invectives. With experience and emotional maturity, you know better. You can talk yourself down from the rage, but you can't deny what happened inside you. In a split second, anger overtook you.

THE PARTS OF ANGER

Consider the components of anger. First, there's the change in body state. Your heart pounds. Your vision narrows. You feel hot. Your stomach clenches. Maybe you feel a heightened sense of mental focus. You go into a state of hyperarousal as your body reacts to a real or perceived threat. This all happens without your control.

Second comes an angry cast of mind, the immediate, automatic intuition at the core of emotion. You've been violated. Your thoughts turn dark. Your mind shifts into high gear, scanning for an enemy.

Third, an object is identified. In emtionally healthy people, anger doesn't just float around unattached. If you feel violated, there's a reason. You might not be objectively right. Maybe you blame the wrong person or jump to some conclusion. In fact, this happens more often than not. But right or not, anger always focuses your attention on some object.

Fourth, you build a story. This is the meaning your mind attaches to what's happened to you. It's not an in-depth explanation, at least not until you think about it for a while. It's just a little protostory. "She's out to get me." "That guy's a jerk." "They're just jealous."

Suppose I'm at home unwinding from a long, draining day. I'm puttering away on some project, when Christina pokes her head around the corner and says, "Were you going to get the kids dinner?" It's a fair question. It doesn't have to mean anything more than the words. She says it in a certain tone of voice, though.

Bam! My body and mind react. I flush. My stomach knots. Thoughts detonate. *Why is she attacking me? Does she think I'm not a good father? Is she saying I don't carry my share of the load?* I feel small. An object comes into focus: my wife's annoying expectations. A story emerges: she doesn't think I'm a supportive husband.

It doesn't matter what Christina meant or what actually happened. I feel violated! I get a certain amount of identity value from being a good dad and husband, so my value feels under attack. The impulse to fight back is strong. If I don't think carefully, what I say next, or the tone of voice I use, won't lead to understanding and greater intimacy. It will lead to more hurt and anger. Perhaps you've experienced something like this.

ANGER IN THE BIBLE

So what does the Bible have to say about all this? A lot ... and most of it isn't good.

Psalm 37:8 says, "Refrain from anger and give up your rage; do not be agitated—it can only bring harm." In Galatians 5, Paul tells us that "outbursts of anger" emerge from the sinful nature. Those who practice anger won't inherit God's kingdom.[4] He puts anger right up there with idolatry, sorcery, and sexual immorality! Proverbs 14:17 says, "A quick-tempered man acts foolishly." A few chapters later, we find this judgment: "A fool gives full vent to his anger."[5]

Not all the Scripture passages about anger are so heavy handed. James 1 directs us to "be quick to hear, slow to speak, and slow to anger, for man's anger does not accomplish God's righteousness."[6] James didn't say, "Quit being angry." He said, "Be slow to become angry." Ephesians 4:26 says, "Be angry and do not sin. Don't let the sun go down on your anger." Scripture is telling us there's a way to be angry without being destructive or sinful. It's possible to experience anger and not have it produce more alienation and brokenness.

Anger becomes a problem when it's held on to and fed. Taking all the verses together, Scripture seems to be saying, "Look, you'll get angry. Face it. Deal with it. Don't let it rule you."

ANGER AND LOVE ALWAYS HOLD HANDS

In the gospel of Mark, we find a story helpful for framing how we think about anger:

> [Jesus] entered the synagogue again, and a man was there who had a paralyzed hand. In order to accuse Him, [the religious leaders] were watching Him closely to see whether He would heal him on the Sabbath. He told the man with the paralyzed hand, "Stand before us." Then He said to them, "Is it lawful on the Sabbath to do what is good or to do what is evil, to save life or to kill?" But they were silent. After looking around at them with anger and sorrow at the hardness of their hearts, He told the man, "Stretch out your hand." So he stretched it out, and his hand was restored.[7]

At this point in the story, the religious leaders were already afraid of Jesus. He was threatening something they loved. Their position? Their authority? Their pride? As Jesus approached the man with the useless hand, they were watching. If Jesus healed the man on the Sabbath, then He was doing forbidden work. It didn't matter that this was restorative work or that it would allow this man to provide for his family. It didn't even matter that it was a miracle! It mattered only whether Jesus was going to keep or break their rule.

Jesus looked at these men, knowing their intention, and stepped into their trap. He asked them a question. Is it lawful—acceptable according to God's law—to do good on the Sabbath? If you picture Jesus with that serene expression from so many paintings, you'd be wrong. The text says Jesus looked at them "with anger and sorrow at the hardness of their hearts." These religious leaders were violating the man's dignity, using him as a pawn in their manipulative scheming.

Jesus loved the man with the crippled hand. Jesus loved to bring freedom and healing to open hearts. These religious leaders were threatening, violating, and obstructing what was precious to Jesus. Jesus felt anger. His anger moved Him to act. But notice this. Even though He felt anger, Jesus didn't violate love. He healed the man, a practical manifestation of God's love. He did this in front of the crowd, inspiring and intriguing people. He spoke to the leaders, not with an attacking tirade but with a simple question meant to pierce their resistance. If they would consider His question, they might begin to think about God in a new way. Jesus felt anger, yet He acted in love.

HEARING THE TRUTH IN YOUR ANGER

Anger is the emotion I wrestle with most. However, as I've learned to listen, my anger has become a capable teacher. Emotions always have truth to tell us. That's how God designed them.

First, anger points out our idols. The Old Testament warns repeatedly about idolatry. In that ancient context, idolatry meant worshipping other gods, bowing down to their idols, keeping their rituals. But this is only the superficial religious exterior of idolatry. The heart of idolatry is to seek our security in something other than

God, allowing it to have governing authority in our lives. Idols are the things we love because they make us feel secure.

Because anger is the emotion we feel when someone or something we love is violated, it's an embarrassingly accurate indicator of where our love lies. The intensity of our anger gauges exactly how much we care about the person or thing that was violated. Steal my scone at the coffee shop? I'll be a bit irritated. Probably confused. I mean, really? It was $2.25. Get your own. But hurt my child, and I'll be enraged.

Anger spins a thread we can follow into the dark maze of our hearts. My own anger has shown that I find value in how much people respect me. When people treat me disrespectfully, I get mad, sometimes disproportionately. For most of my life, this anger focused my attention on the people being disrespectful. But they weren't truly the cause of my anger. The intensity of my anger showed that something precious was being attacked. What did I love this much? Myself, of course. I was angry because these people hadn't paid me the respect I thought I was due.

I keep thinking I'm finding my value in Christ, that I'm no longer a legalist justifying my value to God and the world. Then my anger shows me up. *Nope! Here's another little idol Marc's heart is grasping tightly. See how he loves it?* Anger is a way for God to speak to us about our priorities. Even immature and inappropriate anger.

Second, anger helps us see injustice. Naturally, we see the world selfishly. Our childhood anger is all about us. The first cry of developing anger is "This isn't fair!" Just ask my kids, or yours. They're protesting a perceived injustice. Of course, at first we see only the injustice directed toward us.

As we mature, our ability to see injustice expands to include others. When Jesus shapes our hearts, this accelerates. Jesus came because God loves the world. Paul tells us that there is neither Jew nor Greek, slave nor free, male nor female. Why? Because now we're all one in Christ.[8] Our natural human inclination is to prefer and protect our own group. The gospel teaches us that our own group is *everyone*. That means everyone belongs to us and we belong to everyone else. People different from us are now part of us. Our family. Our children. Our brothers and sisters. When we feel unfairly treated as children, anger erupts. As adults, and maturing followers of Jesus, we should experience a similar kind of anger when we see someone else hurt, taken advantage of, or treated unjustly. That anger should motivate us to do something. Our anger is a flag drawing attention to injustice.

When we learn to listen to our emotions, God can instruct us even when we're dealing with something as difficult as anger. When the motivational energy of anger is aligned with God's character and purpose, it becomes zeal, a passion to protect. As that happens, we experience something mirroring God's experience. It becomes possible for us to feel anger *and respond with love*. Immature anger is almost always selfish, but this changes as we grow and our identity becomes secure in Christ. The more our hearts love what God loves, the more we're able to feel anger and respond with love.

FINDING TRUTH IN JEALOUSY, HATRED, AND WRATH

Three other shades of emotion are often found tangled up with anger—jealousy, hatred, and wrath. They take the blame for so much destruction. They are, we think, the emotional responses of immature, selfish hearts. Mature adults don't feel jealousy, we say. Good people don't hate. Suggest that God experiences these emotions? That's a bridge too far for many. A jealous God, a wrathful God, a God who hates? Aren't those caricatures that religious extremists hold up?

In two decades of ministry, I've had more people than I can count tell me, "I can't worship a God like that." Statements like this reveal something about us and our stories. Our discomfort requires us to engineer ungainly and dishonest interpretations of Scripture that are often self-serving and damaging to others. Yet no matter how uncomfortable an emotion makes us feel, it has truth to teach us.

Here's the truth in jealousy. Jealousy is the emotion you feel when you fear the loss of something you believe you have a rightful claim to.[9] There are two problems with jealousy. First, immature jealousy emerges because of wrong beliefs about what belongs to us. Never forget that essential clause for understanding emotions: "according to your own private logic."[10] Second, immature or hurting people often choose destructive, even dangerous, ways to act on their jealousy. But always keep this distinction in mind: An emotion and the actions a person takes as a result are separate things. The emotion itself isn't bad or sinful; it's not even necessarily immature. The emotion always carries important information. The action is where the problems arise.

Early in my relationship with Christina, I knew I wanted to marry her. We were dating long-distance. At her college, many forces were competing for her heart and time. She was a gymnast surrounded by good-looking athletes; plus, her college friends got to see her every day. I felt jealous. While I didn't have a claim on

Christina—she didn't belong to me—I had hopes for our developing relationship. I feared the loss of our connection. My jealousy carried truth: love is built by spending time together, and time together is a function of proximity. My feelings were saying something true about our circumstances, and that powerful emotion moved me.

I had choices for how I could respond. I could demand that Christina not spend time with these other guys. I could enforce my demand with constant phone calls to check up on her, or with passive aggression or angry outbursts. I could call those guys and threaten them. Jealousy makes actions like these seem reasonable. Instead, I did everything I could to make our time together wonderful. I cooked good food (I'm a much better cook than an athlete). I tried to be as attentive as I knew how. I wanted her to feel safe, loved, and valued when she was with me.

Later Christina decided our relationship was moving too fast and broke up with me. I felt the loss and the threat that we might not get back together. That feeling moved me to act. I wrote and recorded a song for her. I drove four hours to see her and deliver the song expressing my heart. To be sure, jealousy was at play in this, the fear that something threatened our future together. That emotion moved me to protect our relationship and make clear to Christina exactly how much she meant to me.

God's jealousy is something like this, only without flaw or the compromise of sin. God has a rightful claim on our attention and relationship. Our relationship matters to God. When something threatens that relationship, God is moved to act.

Hatred and *wrath* are two other emotional words that can be conversation stoppers. Like anger, they focus our attention sharply on an object. Hatred is the most intense expression of disgust, the emotional response to something we find unacceptable or contaminated. Wrath is the emotional intersection of anger and hatred. These emotions shine a spotlight on something in our world that urgently needs changing.

Because these emotions are so uncomfortable, we feel an aversion to the circumstance or person we believe is causing our pain. That push-away feeling could be as mild as distaste, as visceral as revulsion, or even as fierce as hatred.

Here's a silly example. For a while, I hated the Disney princesses. This strange disdain arose because I was the father of a five-year-old daughter. She loved the princesses beyond comprehension. She wanted to be a princess with a beautiful dress, a castle, a magic carpet, a pet tiger, and a handsome prince. This was probably normal and probably harmless. But my feelings on the subject were sharp.

A few people cautiously suggested that maybe I was being just a bit irrational. I was spending about a thousand dollars of energy on a five-dollar problem. This is always a good indicator it might be time to sit with your emotions and listen. Why so much energy? Where was all this coming from? So I did what all good fathers do: I journaled about Disney princesses. (All dads do that, right?)

I vented about movie plots. I reflected on my daughter's feelings, paying attention to what I felt as I wrote. The Disney princesses seemed to create an image of womanhood I didn't want my children to buy into. I didn't want my daughter to think her value comes from her beauty or to equate the good life with having every desire met. I didn't want her to believe relationship problems can be solved just by wanting it enough or by being more romantic. Most importantly,

I didn't want her to wait around for some square-chinned Prince Charming to rescue her. I wanted *her* to be the hero.

Hatred is the intense inner drive to push away or even destroy something toxic or dangerous. It's been said that hatred isn't the opposite of love; apathy is. *Apathy* means "not caring about something whatsoever." In contrast, both love and hate grow in intensity the more we care about someone or something. Emerson is precious to me beyond words. In my imagination, those princesses were undermining what is unique and invaluable in her. The depth of my love for Emerson resulted in deep antipathy toward the princesses.

After reflecting on this, I calmed down considerably on the subject. I realized I have more influence on my daughter's view of herself than the cartoon characters she likes. They just aren't important enough to warrant hate. But other things are. To hate sex trafficking is appropriate and right. To hate prejudice and racism is godly. To hate when people with power or priviledge rig the system to protect themselves is just. To hate the manipulative use of religion to control people is in alignment with God's heart. Of course, hating my own sin is a step toward spiritual maturity.

As with jealousy, the problem isn't the emotion but the action we take in response. Hate is an emotion of pushing away. We can express it through character assassination, exclusion, rejection, and even violence, but these are choices, not inevitabilities. Even a dark emotion like hate can tell us something true about our hearts and our circumstances.

One of the few scriptures that give us a window into God's hate is Proverbs 6:16–19, which I mentioned earlier:

> The LORD hates six things;
> in fact, seven are detestable to Him:
> arrogant eyes, a lying tongue,
> hands that shed innocent blood,
> a heart that plots wicked schemes,
> feet eager to run to evil,
> a lying witness who gives false testimony,
> and one who stirs up trouble among brothers.

This passage lists some things God sees as toxic, dangerous, and threatening to people. God hates the way we so easily create drama and destruction to get what we want. We lie and scheme; we throw others under the bus. Because God loves us so much, God hates when we harm ourselves and others. God hates injustice!

When we feel this visceral emotional response, we're not broken or sinful. We're feeling something God feels. Sin enters in when our response to the emotion is self-serving, like when we nurture hatred to fortify our own self-righteousness or when it leads us to exclude and destroy others.

"God is love," says 1 John 4:8. Love isn't just one aspect of God's character, coequal with holiness, justice, sovereignty, and whatever other divine qualities you might name. Love isn't something God feels from time to time; it's the summation and fullness of who God is. That means all of God's emotions and actions, even those we don't understand, are rooted in love.

What does this mean for God's hatred or wrath? These are emotional responses rooted in the intensity of love. Chris Tiegreen, in his book *Feeling like God*, puts it like this:

> [Some] question God's wrath, [but] it's really an
> emblem of his love. If he didn't care, he wouldn't
> have it.... His love would be the impotent kind
> that doesn't get upset even when it's abused and
> rejected.... His wrath is controlled.... He doesn't
> fly into a rage, act capriciously, or apply his anger
> unpredictably.... Watering it down may seem
> like an argument in favor of his compassion, but
> it actually weakens our understanding of his love.
> His anger always correlates with his love. Wrath
> is his response to witnessing something he hates,
> and hatred is his response to violations of his love.
> They're all interrelated.[11]

Robert Solomon, one of the foremost theorists on emotion,
made this same point. He said that wrath is the emotion behind
vengeance, and "vengeance is the original passion for justice."[12]
We see hatred and wrath as dark emotions, expressions of an out-
of-control or immature person. But if God is big enough to hold
these emotions without being disrupted or compromised, we have
nothing to fear. God will never be rash or vindictive. The movement
of God's actions will always be toward love. Scripture tells us that
God hates things, that God feels wrath. But before you let those
words scare you off, consider this: If you love someone passionately,
don't you hate anything that threatens or harms him or her?

QUESTIONS FOR REFLECTION

1. What is your experience of anger like? Did anger play a role in your family when you were growing up? How do you relate to anger (in yourself or others) now?

2. How do you understand the apostle Paul's counsel, "Be angry and do not sin"? What does this look like practically?

3. Have you experienced anger as a flag marking injustice? When? What was that experience like?

4. When is our anger most like God's anger? When is it least like God's anger?

Chapter 12

WHEN YOU'RE UNDER THREAT

There are times when fear is good. It must keep
its watchful place at the heart's controls.
Aeschylus, *The Eumenides*

From eternity to eternity the LORD's faithful
love is toward those who fear Him.
Psalm 103:17

Late one Sunday, an announcement broke over network television. It was May 1, 2011. The president broke the news. Osama bin Laden, leader of the al-Qaeda terrorist organization and mastermind of the September 11 attacks was dead. Just hours before, US Army Special Forces had cornered the terrorist leader during a covert mission in Pakistan. All over the United States, enthusiastic, spontaneous celebrations broke out.

A couple of weeks later, I heard a journalist ask a question I'd been pondering. Why was there such a stark difference of reaction between generations? Most of the people at those celebrations were teenagers and young adults. Yet for me and many others my age, the response was more muted. The reporter didn't understand why there was such a noticeable difference.

She interviewed some young people who had been at a demonstration. One college student drilled right down to the core of it. She had been a young child on 9/11. That day was a defining moment for all Americans, but it set the tone for her entire life. Older people called our new reality the "post–9/11 world," a phrase spotlighting the changes we were experiencing. Threat-level colors, removing your shoes at airport security, Internet videos of beheadings—all against the backdrop of a vague, never-ending war.

For those who were adults on 9/11, this was frightening because it was a change from a world that had seemed stable. For this college student and her peers, however, this state of fear was the only reality they knew. They had grown up in a world where one word echoed from every direction: *terror*. Bin Laden became, for them, the face of fear. Killing bin Laden was bigger than homeland security or even primal vengeance. The college student being interviewed said, "He was our real-life Voldemort."[1] A seemingly unstoppable villain from the Harry Potter books, Voldemort was a horrible evil intent on destroying the world. When bin Laden was killed, it was a strike against fear itself.

Fear seems to be a constant presence. The list of all we have to be afraid of gets overwhelming fast. Needles. Dentists. Snakes. Spiders. Confrontation. Public speaking. Violence. Rape. Identity theft. Financial crisis. Cancer. Dying. Environmental catastrophe. Poverty. Being alone. Walking home in the dark. Being trapped in a bad relationship. Not being loved at all.[2] It's fair to characterize the human journey as a struggle with fear.

THE TRUTH IN FEAR

Fear may be the most important emotion for our survival, even if it can be humiliating. Fear keeps us from thoughtlessly walking into dangerous situations. At its most basic, fear is the emotion we feel when we sense danger. The threat may be concrete, like a growling German shepherd blocking the sidewalk. Or it may be abstract, like the fear of failure. The danger may be imagined, like a faceless home invader in the dark, or remembered, like disappointing Mom. Fear can appear as mild anxiety that inflates our stress, or abject terror that paralyzes us.

Despite the discomfort, fear has an important purpose. It stops you in your tracks. In extreme situations, fear gets you to back up and quickly head the other direction. Think of how frequently this emotion has saved you. Maybe fear kept you from getting tangled in a terrible relationship or from making a bad investment. Maybe it stood in your way when you wanted to do something stupid or destructive. Maybe it forced you out of a dangerous situation.

Like anger (and every other emotion), fear is a composite experience. When fear is working right, it goes like this: First, the body reacts to a trigger in the environment or internal state. Just as with anger, breathing accelerates and the heartbeat speeds up. Blood flow is rerouted to the large muscles needed to fight or escape. This quick change in circulation leaves you feeling chilled. You tense up.

Second, anxiety or dread pervades your thoughts. Before your conscious mind can put all the pieces together, you already have an intuition of danger. Quickly your mind homes in on the source of the threat, perceived or actual. It's all you can think about. Urgency to escape builds within you.

Then—even though the time span is often just milliseconds— a protostory explaining all of this emerges in your mind. *I'm going to be exposed and humiliated! I'll lose my house! He's going to kill me!* This sequence happens almost instantaneously, usually outside your control.

This forceful reaction interrupts your normal reasoning processes, causing you to stop. On a sidewalk at night or in a dangerous relationship, this reaction can be lifesaving. But that's not the only time fear shows up. Fear, like all emotions, happens before you have a chance to reflect on your situation. Maybe you identified the wrong object of fear or fixated on something that's not truly dangerous. Maybe the fear you feel in the current moment is rooted in a past experience, as is the case with people who suffer from posttraumatic stress disorder (PTSD). When your fear goes wrong, it keeps you from moving forward when you should.

I must have been nine years old when our paperboy's dog attacked me. I don't remember many details, except the dog seemed enormous. When I spun to escape, he clamped down on my calf. I was sure I was going to be torn apart! Reality wasn't so dramatic. The paperboy called off his dog, and I was left with a nasty bruise and two small puncture wounds that bought me a trip to the doctor, a tetanus shot, and a bowl of ice cream. That was a lifetime ago. Yet nearly four decades later, whenever I hear a dog's guttural growl, primal fear crawls up my spine.

Maybe you've experienced residual fear like this. Our minds build memories and meaning out of associations. That allows old fears to get deeply tangled up in the way we experience the world. Sometimes it's helpful; often it's not. A woman who had an abusive father was right to feel fear of him as a child, but as an adult, it's not helpful for her to fear all the men in her life. Yet that's likely until she deals with the trauma of her childhood.

There is real danger in the world. It's amazing that God gave us the capacity to detect this danger before we have all the facts organized in our conscious minds. This helpful gift can protect us, even keep us alive, but fear can also create a haunting doubt that holds us back from the life God has for us. Sometimes we're afraid of things that aren't really there. In the extreme, a phobia can paralyze us. Other times, this stop-in-your-tracks reflex can obstruct important decisions we need to make. Because fear can keep us from taking action, we miss opportunities. As important as fear is for our safety, it's also one of the most pervasive obstacles to a life well lived. When we learn how to listen carefully to our fear—and more importantly, to what lies behind it—we can find wisdom. Until then, we'll remain reactive, driven by the waves of our fear.

THE BIBLE ON FEAR

Some Christian voices say fear shows a lack of faith. If you feel fear, they say, then you aren't trusting God. Those voices are wrong. When fear functions in a healthy way, it's good and helpful, a God-given gift to keep us out of danger. That's not a sin; it's a blessing, and a path to wisdom.

Scripture confirms that fear is a normal part of life. Words describing fear appear more than 640 times in the Bible.[3] By comparison, the word *heaven* appears 622 times, and the word *love* appears 686 times. In contrast, the word *hell*, which some consider a major biblical doctrine, appears only 15 times. Just 15 times compared with more than 640! In terms of frequency, fear is up there in the big leagues. Nearly every time God or one of God's messengers showed up to interact with someone, the first words in the conversation were something like "Fear not!" Why would God have to start conversations this way? Because we're afraid.

With so many verses encouraging us not to fear, Scripture acknowledges that much of the time we are needlessly afraid. Psalm 23 says, "Even when I go through the darkest valley, I fear no danger, for You are with me."[4] Another psalm tells us, "The LORD is my light and my salvation—whom should I fear?"[5] Isaiah 41:13 says, "I, Yahweh your God, hold your right hand and say to you: Do not fear, I will help you." In 1 Peter, we find this encouragement: "Cast all your anxiety on him because he cares for you."[6] These passages and others tell us we don't have to live controlled by fear. We can find peace even in fearful circumstances.

That's good news. But then the Bible also tells us that sometimes we *should* fear. One psalm tells us, "Happy is the man who fears the LORD, taking great delight in His commands."[7] Another says, "Now the eye of the LORD is on those who fear Him—those who depend on His faithful love."[8] In 1 Peter 2:17, we read this counsel: "Honor everyone. Love the brotherhood. Fear God."

Do you sense a tension? How can the Bible tell us we shouldn't live in fear and, at the same time, tell us to fear God? How does fearing God align with loving God and being loved by God?

AWE AND DREAD: TWO KINDS OF FEAR

I've always struggled with the idea of fearing God. Someone who leads through fear is a bully. If God needs fear to keep us in line, then both love and worship are lies. That's not the picture of the *abba* God that Jesus gave us. Fear is a protective instinct, but a life governed by it isn't good by any measure, nor is it what the New Testament describes as the abundant life.[9]

Yet something about fear is energizing. Roller coasters, horror movies, bungee jumping, extreme sports—these are all experiences of terror. A side of us loves the experience of anticipation, surprise, even dread. In those moments we feel vital and alive. Consider when you're about to experience something big, something that can affect your life enormously. You're suspended briefly between two potential outcomes. Things could go great, or they could go badly. The bungee cord holds, and you're awash in adrenaline, screaming with joy. Or it doesn't, and you're not.

Sometimes this mix of anticipation and suspense is focused on something good. You catch a hint that a surprise birthday party is being thrown for you and a dear friend you haven't seen in years will be there. That welling sense of positive anticipation and wonder is awe.

Those feelings of anticipation and suspense can also be focused on something bad. You open a letter from the IRS, and instead of finding the refund check you expected, it's an invitation to meet with an auditor. When that anticipation is focused on something frightening or intimidating, it's called dread.

In the Old Testament, the word most frequently translated as "fear" is *yare'*.[10] It means "to be afraid, overwhelmed with awe, or astonished." This word encompasses both dread and awe. There's another form of the word, *yir'ah*, which means "to respect, hold in honor, to revere."[11] The same root word takes us to both fear and worship, two experiences that are poles apart. The difference is found in where our focus lies.

Yare' tells us there are things we should be afraid of. The world is a dangerous place. It's right to feel some dread. It even makes sense to feel some dread in regard to our spiritual lives. There are real consequences to pretending we can be God ourselves. Selfishness brings pain, even death, into our lives and the world around us. Some of those consequences affect tomorrow; some shape eternity. Dread seems an appropriate response.

Yet Scripture also tells us God doesn't want us to live governed by fear. Consider 2 Timothy 1:7: "God has not given us a spirit of fearfulness, but one of power, love, and sound judgment." If we're experiencing an ongoing sense of dread, what the apostle Paul calls a "spirit of fearfulness," this likely isn't God's voice. Fear regarding real threats is helpful, the foundation of wisdom. An ongoing dread that hinders faith or joy is just not from God.

When you stand on the lip of the Grand Canyon, you feel *yare'*. It's terrifying! If you lost your footing, the fall would be the end of you. At the same time, the Grand Canyon is so enormous, so beyond us, so beautiful. It's awe inspiring! That's *yir'ah,* what English translations of the Bible stumble so badly in communicating with the phrase "the fear of the Lord."

God is so far beyond us, so holy, so other. God's love is all-encompassing, even when we don't want it, even when feeling known is more painful than hiding. Consider the stunning wonder that God made a way for us to be together forever, at the same time allowing the terrible possibility we might choose the path of separation. When understanding dawns, we worship. This isn't an experience we gather from books and sermons. Descriptions of the Grand Canyon, even pictures, can't possibly convey what we feel when we stand on the rim. Saying we should "fear the Lord" makes no sense until we've stood on the lip of the canyon of God's presence and caught a glimpse of grace.

How can the Bible tell us not to fear but then tell us to fear the Lord? The first appearance of fear in the Bible is in Genesis 3. When humanity violated trust and broke relationship with God, they experienced fear for the first time. They hid. This is where fear leads. We run away. We've been running ever since.

All those passages in the Bible telling us not to fear give a clear reason. They say not to fear, because *God is with us.* When we're in connection with God, when our sense of identity is built on who we are in Christ, so many of our fears can diminish. The object causing our fear may still be there. God often doesn't change our circumstances, but with our value secure in Christ, our priorities shift. Many things that caused us fear before just aren't as important.

This is the truth: You matter. You are loved. A way has been made for you to know and experience God, for you to be with God now and forever. God is so vast, we could remain forever distant. God is so powerful, we could be consumed in an instant. Instead, God holds us close and calls us to relationship, extending grace when we fail. In spite of our weakness, fear, and doubt, God wants us. God wants you. You belong.

Standing on the edge of truth like this, the natural response is awe. That gratitude and wonder is worship. Worship magnifies things. The more we focus on something, the bigger it gets in our perception and the more it occupies our thoughts. When we're in awe of God, we magnify God in our hearts. When we do that, less and less room is available for fear. The *yir'ah* experience of awe solves the *yare'* problem of dread.

That's how the apostle Paul could write these words:

> In all these [difficulties] we are more than victorious through Him who loved us. For I am persuaded that not even death or life, angels or rulers, things present or things to come, hostile powers, height or depth, or any other created thing will have the power to separate us from the love of God that is in Christ Jesus our Lord![12]

Insecurities and fear can occupy so much of our inner world. By God's grace, we need to fear only certain things. Proverbs 19:23 says, "The fear of the LORD leads to life." This is how. When our hearts are filled with awe for God, we have less room for dread. Other fears come into proper perspective.

COMING TO TERMS WITH ANGER AND FEAR

Fear and anger (which we covered in the last chapter) are an emotional pair. They are the push and pull of the same visceral emotional response. When we feel threatened or attacked, we react with one of these emotions. Sometimes anger pushes us forward, and we're intent on stopping the threat. Other times we recoil with fear, sensing we must escape. These emotions course through mind and body, pushing us to change something. The many shades of anger and fear—frustration, rage, wrath, anxiety, dread, and terror—are emotions of discomfort. They often give rise to selfish, reactive choices. We know the turmoil within when these emotions overcome us. It makes sense that we would want to suppress or avoid them.

Yet these emotions, hard as they are, tell us something true. Robert Solomon wrote,

> What characterizes fear and anger and most emotions is their intelligence, their insight, their attunement to the world. Through them, we often get to see and sense what our merely rational minds might ignore, blunder over, or merely rationalize. It is through our fears, our ordinary, normal, reasonable fears, that we rightly recognize that the world is a dangerous place. It is through our anger, our ordinary, normal, reasonable anger, that we rightly recognize that the world is sometimes an infuriating and offensive place.[13]

These hard emotions help us see beyond the calculations of reason. They motivate us to change our circumstances, even to change the world. The danger for us is not in feeling these emotions but in allowing our fear or anger to become disproportionate or reacting in immature, shortsighted, and destructive ways. We want, in our anger or fear, to not sin. Learning to feel and face our hard emotions is a gateway to wisdom. Every shade of fear highlights our perception of a threat. Anger always points us to a perceived violation, perhaps an injustice. With growing emotional and spiritual maturity, we can begin to see when fear or anger is holding us back, or when these visceral responses can move us to act in ways that are good and loving.

The goal of emotional maturity isn't becoming immune to feeling anger or fear. Growing more and more spiritual won't relieve us of these emotions, because they aren't signs of a sin or a flaw or an immaturity. Our goal is to know our identity in Christ and to be able to listen wisely to our emotions, under the influence of the Holy Spirit. Then we can be afraid or angry in the right circumstances in the right proportion with the right people. We can even receive guidance to make godly choices.

If fear is smothering you or anger is overrunning your self-control, something is out of alignment. Some wound in your story is likely amplifying these emotions, leading to overreaction and unnecessary pain. If this is true for you, you may need to ask for help. Tamping down anger or fear through strength of will alone takes enormous effort and nearly always fails over time. You need support. You may need the guidance of an insightful and compassionate counselor. Persistent fear or uncontrollable anger is the tip of an iceberg of pain in your life. You'll need to look beneath the surface. The Holy Spirit is waiting to meet you and help you walk through these dark places. You don't have to live with all-encompassing fear or out-of-control anger. It's God's intention that you would learn from these emotions. That is part of growing in wisdom.

Fear and anger are raw, primal emotions. They often show up as the loudest emotions in our hearts, easiest to pick out from the crowd. In many cases, though, there is another emotion hiding in the shadows. When we lose something we love, we experience sadness. That's where we turn next.

QUESTIONS FOR REFLECTION

1. How would you characterize your experience of fear? Do you consider yourself a fearful person? What impact does anxiety have in your life today?

2. Good and helpful fear alerts you to danger. Unhelpful fear keeps you from moving forward in your life. What are some experiences you've had with fear functioning in these two ways in your life?

3. How do you handle scriptures that tell you to "fear the Lord"? What does that look like in your life practically speaking?

Chapter 13

WHEN YOU WANT, HAVE, AND LOSE

Every heart has its secret sorrows, which the world knows not,
and oftentimes we call a man cold, when he is only sad.
Henry Wadsworth Longfellow, *Hyperion*

Those who mourn are blessed, for they will be comforted.
Matthew 5:4

You've never seen sadness until you've seen my little Emerson when something goes wrong. She and Lucas, her younger brother, were taking turns playing a computer game in our kitchen. They were five and six at the time. In Emerson's mind, her brother had gotten more than his share of time. She reached over to take control of the game. Lucas disagreed with her assessment, pushing her away without taking his eyes off the screen. Her will thwarted, Emerson wound up to give him a good clobber.

I'm generally of the let-them-work-it-out school of parenting, but I don't let them hit each other if I can help it. So I picked up

Emerson and brought her over to my lap. Within moments her anger dissolved into body-shaking sadness. She sat on my lap weeping, shaking as if her little body couldn't contain everything she felt. Periodically she'd throw back her head and wail as though her best friend had just died. It took fifteen minutes for us to get to the place where we could talk.

This wasn't an uncommon experience early in Emerson's life. She feels deeply. As she has grown, she's gotten better at understanding and handling her passion, but the depth of feeling and quick trigger remain. It's easy for me to condescend, to tell her whatever she's sad about isn't a big deal, but I know she's really feeling loss. The scale of our losses has grown since we were kids, but we know how she feels. Sadness—and its most intense expression, grief—are painfully common and universal experiences. Honestly, I don't know many people who haven't had some traumatic loss.

I think of the church family I serve. In just this one small group of people, there's a profound depth of painful experiences. Both parents of one man died from cancer when he was in high school, one shortly after the other. One woman grew up with a single mom. Her parents divorced because her father wouldn't give up his drugs. Several couples carry the wrenching pain of miscarriage. Another woman grew up confused in a home where her depressed mother took desperate measures as she tried to manage her mentally ill husband. Both women and men, more than you would guess, were abused sexually as children. In this room where I gather with my friends every week to worship are people who have lost family, children, jobs, physical ability, even lifelong dreams. If you carry the weight of an enormous loss, you aren't alone.

THE TRUTH IN SADNESS

Sadness is one of the emotions we would rather avoid, poets and blues musicians notwithstanding. When it blows into our lives like unwanted rain, we shelter in social activities, busy projects, comfort food, and Netflix binges. If it catches us, we're left stripped, vulnerable, undone.

Sadness is the feeling you get when you've lost something that matters to you. A complex emotion, sadness includes a yearning for what was lost, a desire for it to be restored, and simultaneous frustration that what was lost is beyond reach. These conflicting feelings grow in sharpness as sadness escalates into grief. Grief seems an infuriating dead end. With anger, there's always hope you can do something about the problem. With fear, you can run away. But when grief overtakes you, there's nothing to do—no handhold, no solution to be found, just a sharp, aching emptiness.

When I was sitting on that front step, overwhelmed by broken love, thinking about driving into a truck, I was feeling grief. I couldn't think. My hope gushed away in uncontrollable sobs. Everything in me wanted to take action, to fix something, but there was nothing to fix. This same emotion came when my dad died. It came again when a couple, both dear friends of mine, experienced infidelity and then divorced. It came again when I realized my own marriage was hanging by a thread and I had put it there. This emotion carries an unbearable truth. We don't get what we want. No matter how skilled or gifted, no matter how smooth our outward appearance, we are only ever fragile, and every good thing can end in a moment.[1]

As much as we'd rather never experience sadness, getting rid of it would be worse. When I began to surface from my depression, the full weight of emotions I'd been ignoring pressed down on me, including waves of sadness. At the time I was meeting regularly with my friend Byron, the trauma therapist.[2] From decades of working with profoundly hurting people, he had learned the vital necessity of sadness. He explained what had happened to me this way: Our capacity for emotional response is like a large window looking out on the circumstances of our lives. This window lets in the full range of emotion from sadness to happiness, but there is a set of heavy drapes with a pull cord to one side. Tug on the cord a little, and the drapes close a bit. Each pull of the cord narrows our view through the window.

When we experience loss or some other hurt, we naturally draw the drapes a bit. We need to lessen the impact of the sadness. Sometimes, in reaction to trauma, we draw the drapes tightly, leaving only a narrow slit of light. We may successfully block out the full pain of sadness, but there is an unintended consequence. The drapes close equally on both ends of the window. When we protect ourselves from grief, we also insulate ourselves from joy. The drapes can become so tightly closed, we're left with only a narrow range of emotions thinly felt and an incomplete view of the world around us. What started as an attempt to make the sadness hurt less ends up numbing our ability to feel anything.

Sadness, for all its pain, is a depth finder for love. We know this intuitively. What happens when someone we know loses a loved one and it seems as if that person isn't grieving all that much? What do we think when we see him or her move on too quickly? We assume something's wrong, even though we can't know the details of that person's grief. Yet we wonder. We instinctively connect the depth of sadness with love.

Kahlil Gibran, the Lebanese poet, wrote, "When you are sorrowful, look again in your heart, and you shall see that in truth you are weeping for that which has been your delight."[3] Emotional theorists say the same thing. Again, Robert Solomon: "The other side of grief, its precondition, is love."[4] If we love, we always live with the possibility of grief.

SADNESS IN THE BIBLE

When it comes to painful moments, the most important thing to know is this: you are not alone. God understands your grief. The Bible describes Jesus as a man who knew grief. Isaiah 53 is a messianic prophecy several New Testament writers quote or allude to in reference to Jesus.[5] "He was despised, and rejected of men; a man of sorrows, and acquainted with grief: and as one from whom men hide their face he was despised; and we esteemed him not."[6]

One example of Jesus' sorrow is at the tomb of Lazarus. As best we can tell, the closest thing Jesus had to a home during His ministry years was in Bethany, a few miles outside Jerusalem. Jesus was close friends with this family—two sisters, Mary and Martha, and their brother, Lazarus. When Lazarus fell sick, the sisters immediately sent word to Jesus. Surely He would heal a friend. But Jesus delayed. Here's what happened when He finally arrived:

> [Jesus] found that Lazarus had already been in the tomb four days. Bethany was near Jerusalem (about

two miles away). Many of the Jews had come to Martha and Mary to comfort them about their brother. As soon as Martha heard that Jesus was coming, she went to meet Him. But Mary remained seated in the house.

Then Martha said to Jesus, "Lord, if You had been here, my brother wouldn't have died."[7]

The sisters were already wrapped up in their grief, feeling the impossible yearning for Lazarus and frustration at how events had unfolded. Martha's words to Jesus sound like part sadness, part accusation. "Lord, if You had been here...." Too many Christian communities blithely teach that someone with true faith will never feel this way.

As I write this, I'm sitting in a friend's home looking out on the Columbia River and the iconic Astoria Bridge. Tamee is known for her endless hospitality and the stunning baked goods that emerge from her welcoming kitchen. This visit, however, took an unexpectedly pastoral turn.

As my family arrived, Tamee and her four children were returning from the funeral of a sixth-grade classmate who had drowned in an unexpected riptide. The family, classmates, and many others from the public-school community had gathered for a memorial service. The local pastor invited to give the eulogy repeatedly told the mourners, "If you are weeping today, you are telling God you don't believe in His power." Perhaps the pastor was trying to make an ill-considered point about God's sovereignty. Practically, though, he was telling a room full of elementary kids they weren't supposed to cry when a friend died. Not only was he being cruel, but he was also contradicting the example of Jesus.

"Lord, if You had been here...." These are painful words of grief and anger that came from a close friend of Jesus. No matter how sturdy your faith, when you experience deep loss, you'll feel grief. There's a solid chance your grief will be expressed through hard words with God. "If only You'd shown up! If only You'd done this one little thing! How could You abandon me?" These aren't prayers uttered with calmly clasped hands. These are raised-fist prayers.

If Jesus had been like that pastor, He would have corrected Martha, maybe even warned her about walking so close to the cliff's edge of doubt. But Jesus didn't chastise the sisters for their questions or reprimand them for their emotional response to painful loss. In Jesus' reaction, we can see clearly: God can handle our pain and hard prayers.

Shortly after He arrived, Jesus, Mary, and Martha went together to Lazarus' tomb. This is the dramatic moment when Jesus got to prove who He was, and the hopes of humanity were confirmed. He stood in front of the tomb, God-made-flesh face-to-face with death, our inexorable enemy. If this had been a movie, the camera would have zoomed in. The music would have swelled, building to a crescendo.

What wonder do we see next? Read it yourself in John 11:35:

Jesus wept.

That's it. Don't rush past this revelation. We expect God to beat death, with Lazarus mummy-shuffling from the tomb. What we don't expect is God weeping. Here was Jesus, standing in front of the grave of a close friend, responding exactly as you or I would—feeling sorrow, crying for His friend.

Yes, Lazarus would soon be raised from death. But even though the story moves on, don't move on too quickly. The image of Jesus crying at the graveside of a friend is a paradigm buster. First, grief isn't wrong. Jesus wept, and Jesus was without sin. It's not a defect in your character. It's not a lack of trust in God. It's the normal and right response to loss. Second, God knows how grief feels. Jesus is not only the full revelation of the Father to us; He is also God's firsthand experience of being human. What Jesus felt, God knows.

Your sadness will make you feel alone, sure that no one understands what you're going through. That's normal, but it's not true. You are held by one who knows what you lost and how it felt. You aren't alone in that dark graveside garden of pain.

HOW CAN YOU BEST HELP A GRIEVING PERSON?

Grieving people, as well as their friends and family, frequently ask this question: How long should you grieve?

The best explanation I've ever heard came from Steven, the former pastor so vital in my early recovery.[8] When you're in the bathroom doing your business, how do you know when you're done? You just know, right? You're done when it's all out. That's the same way you know how long to grieve. You grieve until it's all out. No one else can tell you how long that will be. They don't know; only you do.

You can't let people, social convention, or relational discomfort get in the way. You grieve until you're done. You might even find that same grief surfacing again later.

The analogy is instructive on many levels. What happens if you need to go to the bathroom and you don't? It causes stress, even pain. If you hold off for too long, you'll get sick. That's true with grieving too. People who haven't dealt with their grief get sick. Untended grief shapes their emotional experience and thoughts. For some, it manifests as anger, even rage. For others, it settles into depression. Many show physical symptoms like severe fatigue or ulcers. The stress of grief compromises our immune system as well, opening the door for all kinds of infectious diseases—especially for older people.[9] Learning how to grieve is one of the best things we can do for our emotional and spiritual health.

Our culture tells us we should grieve only so long and in certain appropriate ways. We're uncomfortable when grief floods over these boundaries. Think about the ways we often comfort others. We pat them on the back. We tell them everything will be okay. We encourage them not to cry. But for someone grieving a great loss, everything is *not all right*. Life has been irreparably changed. It may be better eventually, but today grief is telling the truth: everything is not okay. In regard to this particular loss, life will not be all right again. When we tell people not to cry, we're asking them to create an outward illusion of peace betraying their inward reality of pain. We're asking them to lie.

When those you care about are grieving, sit with them. Affirm that their feelings are true and right and important. Encourage their tears. Give them whatever space and time they need. When we don't, we're usually protecting ourselves from discomfort by managing their emotions. That's not fair. It's not healthy either—and it probably points to untended pain in our own lives.

Unfortunately, Christians are just about the worst at this. Not only do we have the same discomfort with grief everyone else has, but we also have a backpack full of encouraging words we feel obliged to share. Grieving people often say things that are theologically incorrect, and some of us feel an urgency to correct them on the spot. Sometimes it seems that the loss they're feeling is a consequence of bad behavior, and some of us think perhaps we can help them grow by pointing that out. Or maybe in an effort to encourage them, we start quoting Bible verses about God drying every tear and sorrow being no more. None of this is helpful.

Joseph Bayly experienced the death of three children. Many parents have children die, but as a writer and publisher, Mr. Bayly was able to share his experience. In his book *The View from a Hearse*, he wrote,

> I was sitting, torn by grief. Someone came and talked to me of God's dealings, of why it happened, of hope beyond the grave. He talked constantly, he said things I knew were true.
>
> I was unmoved, except to wish he'd go away. He finally did.
>
> Another came and sat beside me. He didn't talk. He didn't ask leading questions. He just sat beside me for an hour and more, listened when I said something, answered briefly, prayed simply, left.
>
> I was moved. I was comforted. I hated to see him go.[10]

Almost every grieving person I've ever talked to feels the same way. I know I did. Don't comment. Don't preach. Don't encourage. Just be with. The Bible gives direct guidance to us on this point. Paul wrote, "Rejoice with those who rejoice; weep with those who weep."[11] That's clear, isn't it? If someone in your life is mourning, the loving thing is not to get the person to stop crying. The loving thing is to simply be there, quietly sharing in the pain. At some point the grieving will be done. Then your encouragement will be needed.

WHAT IF YOU'RE THE ONE GRIEVING?

If you've experienced loss, whether from the death of someone you love, the death of a relationship, or any other kind of loss, you'll experience grief. You're not flawed or weak. Those feelings are the fraying break in the rope of relationship you've built over time. They represent the depth of love and experience you shared. To minimize those feelings, to hide from them or deny them, is to dishonor the relationship you had and the impact it had on your life.

Grief is a natural process that takes the time it takes. Our culture wants to rush grief, to skirt around it. Resist that pressure. Trying to shortcut grief always leaves a mark. Displaced and disproportionate anger, a cynical or bitter spirit, even some kinds of persistent fears are the emotional scars of unprocessed grief.

First, allow yourself to feel the full weight of your sadness. You may not want to. Sadness may leave you feeling vulnerable, ugly, like an outsider when everyone else seems to be busily enjoying life. But you must face it. Your grief contains many losses, each of which must be tended to, a collection spanning the reach of your life together.

You've lost companionship. You've lost the shared story you were building. You've lost hopes and dreams. You've lost the opportunity to continue whatever conversations were in process. Maybe you've lost the chance to be reconciled. Your grief is a mosaic made from many shards.

My mom and dad had been married for almost seventeen years when Dad died unexpectedly. Of course Mom grieved profoundly. What was surprising, though, were the many small losses contained in the larger loss. Some seemed almost trivial. Who would take out the trash now? Who would reach the highest kitchen shelves? Each was a symbol of a deeper pain. Once, my mom told me the thing she was angriest about during her grief was how little Dad had shared the family finances with her. He paid the bills. He filed the paperwork. It didn't occur to her until it was too late that there was crucial information she needed. She spent sad, frustrated hours digging through his files, looking for insurance documents, banking documents, all necessary for carrying on with life. More than once, she pounded her fist on the table, demanding God bring Dad back for just an hour so he could tell her where all those important documents were.

Fully processing your grief means owning these many facets. As much as you would rather not, you must think about these losses and feel the sadness. Journal about them, bringing to memory both the good and bad of each facet of your relationship with this person. Talk your feelings through with a trusted friend or counselor who will simply be present and listen, a witness to your grief.

Second, allow yourself the time you need. One of the functions of grief is that you are reimagining your life in light of the loss. There is simply no shortcut. Like the transition of winter into spring, this process requires whatever amount of time it requires. If you don't give yourself the time you need, the grief will continue to bleed out into your life and relationships, even if you don't want it to.

Third, as you grieve, give yourself grace. Your life has been interrupted. The grief will show up in your body and mind. At times your memory will fail you. At inopportune moments, you'll feel overcome with vivid memories. You'll be tired, because grief is hard work. You won't be as productive as you were before. Your mind will wander. You'll experience waves of emotion, sometimes in ways that seem irrational. You'll experience flashes of anger, envy at the relationships others have, and shame for feelings you think you shouldn't feel. Through all of this, sadness like the tide will wash over you again and again, only to recede each time. All of this is normal. The emotional process of grieving is how you integrate the loss into your personal story.

Now most of what I've written here speaks to someone whose friend or family member has died. While that's an obvious kind of trauma, many other experiences elicit grief. When we don't process those losses, the grief ends up corrupting our emotions and experiences, even years later.

A friend of mine got married many years ago, with clear hopes for the future. He thought things were going to be one way, but life turned out differently. He didn't lose a person to death; he lost a dream of what he hoped his marriage would be like. Over years this unprocessed pain grew into bitterness toward his spouse. That bitterness infected his attitude and words, causing enormous damage. The resentment was a scab over the loss of a dream he had never processed. He wasn't able to change the tone of his marriage until he grieved the loss of that original dream.

When someone dies, we know we need to grieve. But when our hopes and dreams fail, we need to grieve that too. A child born with a disability, a business failure, a spouse who develops mental illness, an experience of abuse—these all involve the death of a dream. In every case, we need to grieve.

Grief is common to all of us, yet we're the children of a culture that avoids grief like sunbathers running from the rain. This natural process of grieving has become alien to us. You'll want to run from it, but it's best for your heart to push into it. Journal. Take frustrated walks with lots of tears. Write blues songs. Paint angry, abstract pictures. Do what you need to do. Grieve until you're done. You may find you need a trail guide to assist you in navigating the path. Start with compassionate friends who are willing to be with you, bearing no urgency to see you fixed or better. Seek out a good counselor. When you're ready, you may find some recommended books helpful as well.[12]

A REMINDER OF ETERNITY

Grief is unique among emotions. Love builds the bonds of intimate relationships. Fear protects us from danger. Anger moves us to act against injustice. These emotions move us in a clear direction we can act on. There is less certainty with grief. Some theorists suggest grief's purpose is to reinforce our bonds with family. Others suggest it's meant to draw a community together. All our other emotions move us to do something, to take some kind of action, but grief often paralyzes us, leaving us vulnerable. What purpose could that serve?

It's strange that one of our most powerful emotions seems to make so little sense. It's been called the irrational emotion.[13] We are relational creatures. We find our sense of self in our relationships with others and with God. Losing precious people shakes us to our core. The pain we feel is like the breaking of our own self. Grief elicits the desire for what was lost to be restored, but if this world is all there is, that feeling is a cruel hoax. Everyone dies. In a purely material world, death should be the least surprising outcome. The only posture that makes sense is acceptance, yet every time we experience death, it comes to us as an intruder, an invader. Everything in us rebels against it.

But what if this near-universal experience of grief is telling us something important? If the story told in the Bible is true—that we were created for life and relationships without end—then perhaps instead of being an irrational desire, our grief is a bright window into reality. The violent tearing of grief and its residual ache tell us the truth. Death feels wrong and unfair because it is. Our grief is a kind of knowing, a deep insight that goes beyond what we can see and measure. We know, at the level of cells and brain chemicals and intuition, that we were made for eternity.[14]

Grief tells us the truth of our current reality. We have lost something important. That loss is painful and disorienting. The stories we were planning now must be rewritten. People die. Dreams die. We lose things important to us. Yet our grief points us toward another truth. God brings life where there once was death. Relationships were designed to last forever. Death is coming to an end. We experience grief today, but we experience it because we know in our very being that this isn't what we were made for.

In the moment of our grief, we are not alone. God knows our pain and loss and walks with us in that crushing circumstance. The psalmist captured the work that happens in our hearts as we face our grief: "He heals the brokenhearted and binds up their wounds."[15] But a time is coming when all our grief will finally be resolved and our yearning will be fulfilled. Our intense grief reminds us, "He will wipe away every tear from their eyes. Death will no longer exist; grief, crying, and pain will exist no longer, because the previous things have passed away."[16]

That sounds very much like happiness, and this is the emotion we turn to next.

QUESTIONS FOR REFLECTION

1. Think about your most painful experiences of grief. What were you grieving? How did your grief reflect on that lost relationship or object?

2. Would you say you're more of a feeler or more of a denier when it comes to grief and loss? Do you primarily push into the grief and feel it, or do you push away from the grief with denial or distraction? Why do you think you do this?

3. Think of the person who has been the most helpful to you in the face of grief. What did that person do for you? How did that help you?

4. How does it affect you knowing that Jesus experienced great loss and grief?

Chapter 14

WHEN YOU'VE GOT WHAT YOU WANT

If you make up your mind not to be happy there's no
reason why you shouldn't have a fairly good time.
Edith Wharton, "The Last Asset"

I know that there is nothing better for them than to rejoice
and enjoy the good life. It is also the gift of God whenever
anyone eats, drinks, and enjoys all his efforts.
Ecclesiastes 3:12–13

Happiness seems to be the holy grail of the emotional life. As I'm writing this, Amazon.com lists more than ninety thousand titles on the subject. There's a whole subcategory called "Happiness Self-Help," with 25,000 titles. If you read one of those books every day, you would be reading for almost fifty years! Where how-to books don't cut it, we're turning to life coaches and therapists, support groups and antidepressant medications in record numbers. An awful lot of people aren't happy but wish they were.

For a while, Christina and I watched *The Voice*, a musical competition show. It was similar to *American Idol*, the biggest, most well-known show of the genre. But *The Voice* was different in a significant way: the judges sat with their backs to the singer. Their first impression was based on voice alone. For an industry obsessed with appearance, that change was revolutionary.

In one episode I recall, I was struck by the contestant's "green-room interview" before taking the stage. As I remember, she lived in Nashville, Tennessee, worked successfully as a backup singer, and regularly toured with world-class acts. As a songwriter living in Nashville, she had the opportunity to collaborate with talented professionals. She had already cowritten a couple of hit songs. By any reasonable definition, she was successful.

Yet as she stood in the wings about to sing for the judges, she was nearly in tears. "This is my chance!" she said. "It's my turn to come out of the shadows and get the recognition I deserve. This means more to me than anything." In spite of already making a living doing what she loved, she wasn't happy.

Isn't this how we often pursue happiness? No matter what we already have, we want something more or different. I've heard the same kind of comment from so many.

> If I could just have another baby …
> If I could just get this job …
> If I could just get more people to hear my music …
> If I could just marry her …
> If I could just catch a break financially …

We believe if we could just walk through a door into different circumstances, everything would be better. We would be satisfied. We could finally be happy.

WHAT IS HAPPINESS, REALLY?

For something we spend our lives chasing, happiness is notoriously difficult to pin down. Among therapists, psychologists, life coaches, and preachers, there is quite a bit of debate as to whether happiness is an emotion or something else. Some have suggested that happiness is an attitude. Others say it's a choice we make to accept our current circumstances. Does happiness happen because of our external circumstances or our internal experience? Is it emotion or something else? Even the dictionary seems caught in the same dilemma. Here are two of the primary meanings *Merriam-Webster* gives for the word *happy*: "favored by luck or fortune" and "enjoying or characterized by well-being and contentment."[1]

The first definition portrays happiness as something that happens to us, built from the blocks of good circumstance. Many pursue happiness this way. That backup vocalist certainly did. If good things happen to us, then we can be happy. The second definition is more ambiguous. If we're content, is it because our circumstances are agreeable and we have everything we need? Or are we content because we've learned some emotional or spiritual skill enabling us to be content regardless of circumstances? Is happiness simply a trick of perception? There's a shade of East-West tension embedded here. The voices of our Puritan forebears tell us if we work hard, we'll find satisfaction; Zen Buddhists caution that happiness is found only by accepting what is.

Modern Western culture leans toward the first definition. If good things are happening to us, we expect to feel satisfied. Want happiness? Increase your good circumstances and get rid of your unfortunate ones. Walk into your boss' office and say with authority, "You, sir, are an unfortunate circumstance! I quit!" Then walk out in search of fortunate circumstances. Perhaps invest in winning the lottery or, more reasonably, find a better job you enjoy. Pursue your dream!

This is the modern path to happiness, the self-evident quest enshrined in the Declaration of Independence. All of us ought to be free to pursue our own happiness, right? But do we even know what exactly we're pursuing? Better circumstances? A more peaceful interior life?

Those who suggest that happiness comes from external circumstances are telling part of the truth. Those who tell us happiness is an inside job, rooted in attitude, are also telling part of the truth. This same tension is present in every emotion. All emotions are responses to some kind of object, often external to us. Yet our assessment of that object draws on our life experience, our expectations, and the stories we construct to make sense of what is going on.

This tension is far more obvious with happiness. Why? Because happiness is the emotional state we long for. Not many set out in pursuit of anger or grief. Because no one is interested in learning how to have more anger or grief, there is no controversy about where those emotions come from. But happiness? That's the emotion we're willing to do nearly anything to find. Every religion, worldview, and therapeutic modality offer their suggestions.

To be clear, happiness *is* an emotion. It's so much more obvious when happiness hits us with intensity. In those moments we call the emotional response we're having joy or ecstasy. Those feelings burst in on us, sparkling and vibrant, sometimes so overwhelming we laugh involuntarily or cry. But happiness can also be very subtle, something we miss if we're not paying attention.

The reason happiness can be so easy to overlook, even misunderstand, is that the motivation happiness provides is different from other emotions. Fear and anger, even in their lowest intensities, are emotional responses pushing us to act. There's a threat or violation; something in our circumstances needs to change. Happiness is just the opposite. It's the emotional response to having what we need or want, the feeling that comes when things are just right.

We've all had that transcendent moment when these words come spontaneously: "Wow! I wish this would never end." Maybe we're sitting on a beach at sunset. The temperature and light breeze are perfect. Maybe we're cuddling by the fire with a loved one. A sense of satisfaction blossoms within us. It's strange to call this feeling a longing, but it is—a longing for this very moment to continue forever.

Happiness is the emotional response of having, holding, finding. Instead of moving us to change our circumstances, happiness motivates us to keep things as they are for as long as possible. We have, at least for a moment, satisfaction. We're not chemically and physiologically ramped up in fight or flight. We're peaceful. The body's complex system for maintaining homeostasis is working. We're awash in the brain chemicals of well-being. In this very moment, we have what we need. Or what we think we need. Most simply, happiness is the emotion of contentment. Even the more exuberant expressions of happiness, like joy and ecstasy, are essentially powerful experiences of the perfect moment. Our hearts cry out, "This! Right here, right now. This is what I want more of."

I suspect this is one reason why happiness is so hard to find for people who struggle to be present—conscious and aware of what is going on within them in the moment. At least that's been my experience. For most of my adult life, my mind was somewhere other than here and now. With so much of my value tied up in my performance, my thoughts were always preoccupied. There were always past moments of failure to rehash. If I ran out of those, I could worry about the future. With all this regret and worry, my mind was rarely able to quietly enjoy the present moment. Not coincidentally, I rarely felt happy. Even if my circumstances were positive, my inner world was anxious and agitated, untangling the next problem.

At the core, happiness arises when we find what we need to survive—food, shelter, and belonging. But humans are complex creatures, and what comprises well-being for us is also complex: a sense of purpose rather than aimlessness; meaningful autonomy rather than bondage; acceptance rather than shame or rejection; personal growth rather than stagnation; a sense of place and belonging rather than alienation. Not to mention the sense of peace or contentment we can find spiritually. For most of us, qualities like these dramatically influence our sense of well-being and satisfaction with life.[2]

Yet even among these qualities, different people have different preferred values. Some people see autonomy as central to their happiness. They will sacrifice a sense of belonging and social approval so they can make their own choices when and how they want. Others view belonging as the highest value and identify as being happy even though the group they belong to restricts their autonomy and personal growth. To complicate matters even further, our personal stories deeply influence our sense of what feels right. We can have an emotional response of contentment to things that have worked for us in the past, even though they're objectively destructive. And of course euphoria can masquerade as happiness for a while, even the kind manufactured by addictive substances or adrenaline.

Once again we find our emotional responses are telling us the truth about something in our lives and circumstances. Within our experience of happiness, we hear this message: In this moment we have what we need. Or possibly what we think we need. But as is so often the case with emotion, we can miss this information or misinterpret it. So when we're unhappy, we very often draw the wrong conclusion about who or what is to blame. That's why our most common path to happiness is attempting to change our circumstances.

DOESN'T GOD WANT US TO BE HAPPY?

We're so deeply committed to our quest for happiness that we often enlist God in our project. Listen to religious people talk about the choices they want to make. Perhaps they're in tough or painful circumstances, thinking about making a change—maybe changing jobs, moving, getting married, or getting divorced. There are reasons not to move forward, but desire often conscripts reason to its cause. At some point they'll likely say, "God just wants me to be happy, right?"

It's a hard premise to disagree with on its face. God is love. God is a perfect parent. We know that "all things work together for the

good of those who love God."[3] Psalm 37:4 says that God will give us
the desires of our hearts. So if our hearts desire happiness, isn't that
what God wants for us too? I certainly don't think God is opposed to
our happiness. God isn't peering down over a ledger, hoping to upset
our plans just to teach us a lesson. Yet Scripture suggests that God
sees happiness differently from the way we do.

In the Old Testament, one word often gets translated "happy"
or "happiness." It's the Hebrew word *esher*. Likewise, a single Greek
word, *makarios*, is rendered "happy."[4] Both words are translated
"happy," but both can also be translated "blessed." Most every time
you see the word *blessed* in English, you can substitute *happy*, and the
other way around.

A quick review of a handful of passages where *esher* is found
shows that either translation works well. Psalm 32:1 (NIV) says,
"Blessed is the one whose transgressions are forgiven, whose sins are
covered." Psalm 40:4 (NIV) tells us, "Blessed is the one who trusts in
the LORD, who does not look to the proud, to those who turn aside
to false gods." Proverbs 3:13 (NIV) says, "Blessed are those who find
wisdom, those who gain understanding." Substitute *happy* for *blessed*
in all these verses, and they sound right and true.[5]

There are, however, a number of places where the Bible talks
about people being blessed in ways that don't sound happy at all.
One example? The Beatitudes in Matthew: "Blessed are the poor in
spirit, for theirs is the kingdom of heaven. Blessed are those who
mourn, for they will be comforted. Blessed are the meek, for they
will inherit the earth."[6] It's hard to read *happy* for *blessed* in those
verses. Happy are the poor in spirit? Happy are those who mourn?
Happy are the meek? Isn't that a contradiction?

The book of James says, "Consider it a great joy, my brothers, whenever you experience various trials, knowing that the testing of your faith produces endurance."[7] Joy in the face of trials? That doesn't sound like happiness at all. The apostle Paul wrote, "I have learned to be content in whatever circumstances I am. I know both how to have a little, and I know how to have a lot. In any and all circumstances I have learned the secret of being content— whether well fed or hungry, whether in abundance or in need."[8] Here contentment is unhitched from circumstances. Paul's secret? "I am able to do all things through [Christ] who strengthens me."[9] If this is the kind of happiness God wants for us, there's little to suggest it includes having circumstances go our way. When people say, "God just wants me to be happy," I don't think this is what they mean.

In our culture, happiness is about feeling contentment because circumstances are going our way. However you slice it, that's not what Scripture says happiness is. If that's not what happiness is, then you certainly can't find happiness by chasing better circumstances. According to Scripture, happiness is possible for people in terrible circumstances. Wealth, position, and fame can't guarantee it. Happiness can come just as easily from God disciplining us as from God bringing pleasant things into our lives. If happiness is the emotion of having what we need, perhaps we struggle so hard with being happy because we don't understand what we truly need.

Does God want us to be happy? Sure, but it doesn't seem to be God's first concern for our lives. God wants us to be holy.[10] God wants us to do justice and love mercy.[11] God wants us to be forgiven[12] and to be forgivers.[13] God wants us to grow in the evidence of the Holy Spirit's work in our lives and show deeper "love, joy, peace, patience, kindness, goodness, faith, gentleness, [and] self-control."[14] God wants us to mature in the image of Christ.[15] These things matter to God and are what God is working to bring about in our lives.

YOU CAN'T GET THERE FROM HERE

It seems happiness is a side effect that comes when we experience all these other things God intends for us. That's the trick with happiness: it can't be directly pursued. The philosopher Eric Hoffer commented wryly, "The search for happiness is one of the chief sources of unhappiness."[16] In the same way, unhappiness is also a side effect, not necessarily connected to outward circumstances. No one ever became unhappy by pursuing unhappiness. We've all heard stories of wealthy, famous, or influential people who are profoundly unhappy. We know people who have gotten exactly what they set out to find and are still miserable to be around. When we pursue happiness, we find ourselves in a never-ending race trying to cross a finish line that's always just beyond our reach. Why is this? The source of our unhappiness isn't outside us.

We change our circumstances in the hope of finding happiness and then show up with the same old stories that were making us unhappy to begin with. If our hearts are full of bitterness and unforgiveness, new scenery won't change that. More money won't lift crushing shame. If we have a broken sense of identity or carry painful wounds from trauma, a change in circumstances can give us some momentary peace or reestablish safety, but it cannot mend wounds within us.

How then can we find happiness? One of the oft-quoted scriptures on the subject is Psalm 37. Here we find the incredible promise that God will give us the desires of our hearts. The passage is mostly misquoted and taken out of context. Yet there is real wisdom if we step back from the bumper-sticker version. "Do not be agitated by evildoers," it begins. "Do not envy those who do wrong. For they wither quickly like grass and wilt like tender green plants."[17]

That first instruction covers so many of the reasons we find ourselves unhappy. We fret. Our hearts become agitated when life doesn't go our way. When life is uncomfortable, we get anxious. People out there do bad things, sometimes to us. We see all of this, and we worry. We also envy. We look at other people—at what they have, what they look like, how their lives are going—and we wish our circumstances were like theirs. These things occupy our attention, but they're temporary, like withering grass. Worse yet, worry and envy leave no space for contentment. Envy and contentment can't share the same heart.

Instead of focusing on what's bad in the world or on what we don't have, Psalm 37 tells us to focus somewhere else: "Trust in the LORD and do what is good; dwell in the land and live securely."[18] When we trust God, we can let go of our need for circumstances to be perfect. When we focus on doing good, our vision shifts away from what causes us to worry and envy. Only then does the psalm come around to its famous promise: "Take delight in the LORD, and He will give you your heart's desires."[19]

God actually promises to give you the desires of your heart. But look closely. God isn't promising to change your circumstances. This isn't a free pass to Disney World and a pony. A heart full of worry desires safety. A heart full of envy desires what it doesn't have. In contrast, a heart focused on trusting God desires more of God and what God wants. This is a heart that delights in God. When you delight in God, God can unreservedly fulfill this promise. God will give you your heart's desire. God will give you God's own self.

If I'm unhappy because my sense of identity is broken, what I need is to know and experience my true identity in Christ. If I'm unhappy because I have no motivating sense of purpose or passion, what I need is to pursue God's heart. As I mature in the likeness of Jesus, I will more frequently experience the purpose and passion of God. If I'm unhappy because of emotional brokenness or untended trauma in my story, what I need is healing. This can happen as I give God more and more access to my heart and God leads me to healing people.

When people say, "God just wants me to be happy," what they usually mean is "I believe this certain thing will make me happy. Because God loves me, God must want me to have this certain thing too." That's nothing more than projection. They're assigning their own desires to God. Instead, Psalm 37, taken as a whole, offers a different script: "I want to be happy, and I believe God knows best what will make me happy. Because I trust God, I want whatever God wants for me." As we focus on God, our desires become more like God's desires. As we desire what God desires, our wills come into alignment with God's will. When our wills are in alignment with

God's will, we get what we want. Why? Because we finally want what God wants.

In this passage and others like it, Scripture suggests that if we set our minds on God and God's ways, happiness—contentment and blessedness—will come as a result. Instead of chasing circumstances we hope will make us happy, we pursue more important goals—intimacy with God, authentic relationships with others, compassion and justice for those around us. When we find our delight in these things, then we will be happy. *Blessed* may be a better word.

There is one last emotion we'll examine. It's likely the most important, since it's the emotion that moves us toward godly behavior more than anything else. In fact, this emotion puts our hearts most closely in alignment with God's heart.

QUESTIONS FOR REFLECTION

1. The dictionary presents two different viewpoints on being happy: "favored by luck or fortune" and "enjoying or characterized by well-being and contentment." Where does your personal definition for *happiness* fall? How have you seen this play out in your life?

2. If happiness is the emotion of contentment, then central to experiencing happiness would be the ability to be truly present in the moment. How are you when it comes to noticing what is really happening in your inner landscape and outer circumstances? If you struggle with being present, why do you think this is?

3. In both the Old Testament Hebrew and the New Testament Greek, the words *happy* and *blessed* are generally interchangeable. How might these two concepts be related?

4. Psalm 37 says that God wants to give us the desires of our hearts but indicates that this promise is activated for us when our hearts desire God. What does this say to you about the nature of happiness?

Chapter 15

WHEN YOU FEEL LIKE GOD

Compassion asks us to go where it hurts, to enter into places of pain, to share in brokenness, fear, confusion, and anguish.... Compassion means full immersion in the condition of being human.

Henri Nouwen, Donald McNeill, and Douglas Morrison, *Compassion*[1]

I give you a new command: Love one another.

John 13:34

I love words and everything about them—their historical development, their shades of meaning, the many ways they can be creatively woven together. I love reading and playing with words. It's not surprising that I love writing. Most of all, I love that words have specific meanings. Placeholders like *stuff*, *thing*, and *great* are ingredients for a bland, colorless word broth. But words with focus? I love those. Words like *verisimilitude*. That word refers to something that appears true. *Acquiesce* is another favorite. It means "to give up quietly." The word fades away, like someone backing out of an argument.

I don't love when words get used incorrectly. I get a tiny bit irritated when people say "literally" when they mean "really, truly." My hackles go up when someone says something is "not fair" but means something is "not going my way." Fairness isn't about you or me; it's about equity.

As much as I wish it weren't true, words have a problem. They get watered down. As people use words in new and different situations, definitions shift. *Awesome* used to mean "terrible." Something awesome was big, overwhelming, and terrifying. Today *awesome* just means "great," and *great* doesn't mean anything. *Sorry* used to mean "sorrowful," as in "I feel sorrowful about how I hurt you." Not anymore. Now it's a throwaway word, the beginning of an excuse: "I'm sorry you feel that way, but...." All the sorrow has been drained away.

Chief among watery words is *love*. It's the most enrapturing experience of life; it's also how I feel about Ben & Jerry's Cherry Garcia ice cream. It's become a featureless stand-in for almost any positive feeling. This drift of meaning is a problem because *love* is an important word, a concept crucial for relationships, family, emotional health, and our relationship with God.

We've heard that God loves everyone, but if we're not clear what love means, what does this statement actually say? God thinks nice thoughts about us? God likes us the way we like chocolate? Factor in our baggage and uncertainty about whether it's okay for God to have emotions, and our confusion grows thick. If the Bible says God loves people yet God doesn't really have emotions, what does that mean?

THE PROBLEM WITH *AGAPE*

If you've sat through more than a year's worth of sermons, you've undoubtedly heard about the word *love* in the Bible. When the New Testament was written, Greek had four words for love: *philia, eros, storge,* and *agape. Philia* was family or brotherly love. *Eros* was romantic, idealistic love. *Storge* was affection—those kind, gentle feelings we have toward people we like. Then there was *agape,* a committed, deep care for someone.

The writers of the New Testament never used *eros* or *storge.* They used only *philia* and *agape.* When they used *agape,* they remodeled the cultural meaning into something more powerful. When John defined God as love, this is the word he used.[2] God *is agape.* When we're told God so loved the world that God sent Jesus, the word is the verb form of *agape.*[3] When Paul defined love in 1 Corinthians 13—"love is patient, love is kind. Love … does not keep a record of wrongs"—that was all *agape.*[4] Through its use in the New Testament, *agape* came to represent the highest and best picture of love, love that cares for another's best interests, acts on that person's behalf, and gives itself away.

Two thousand years later, it's the name of a muffler shop, a carpet-cleaning service, and a company that makes herbal supplements for cleansing your colon. Talk about definition drift! *Agape* has deeper problems, though. It's been installed on a pedestal, displayed in the theology library, where only pastors and seminary professors have access to it. *Agape* is the love of God. That's a big deal. God loves perfectly. God even loves enemies and rebels! This kind of love seems completely out of reach. A few resulting ideas about *agape* have crept into our minds, ideas that just aren't true.

The first myth is that *agape* is "Christian love." We're told in 1 John 4 that God is love, and love comes from God.[5] Just a few verses later, we hear that when we love, God's love is perfected in us.[6] Some preachers leap from these verses, saying because only Christians, who have accepted Jesus, have God in them, only Christian love is truly unselfish, other centered, like God's. This isn't what the text says at all.

These verses say God is love and all love comes from God. All love—even in sinful or broken people, even in those we disagree with. Love, wherever it's found, is a mirror reminding us we were created in God's image. All of us! We twist that image with pride, fear, insecurity, and sin. That's true, but at the core, love exists because of God. These verses hint that maybe God can be found in more places than we expect.

The second myth is that *agape* is only intellectual, an abstract principle. "Of course I love everyone," one Christian says. "I don't hate anyone. I think all people are valuable." Words like these are a statement of belief, but are they loving? Sometimes words like these follow remarkably insensitive or demeaning statements of judgment. In that moment the words become a self-justifying smoke screen. An abstract *agape* that never shows up in real action toward real people is really no love at all.

God created humanity, so every human has essential dignity. Followers of Jesus are called to love everyone, even enemies— explicitly our enemies. That's hard to do.[7] I don't feel affection for people who hurt me, nor do I feel drawn to serve those who hate me. The escape hatch is to relegate *agape* to the heady realm of abstract ideals—something to live up to, to hold out as a goal, but something we can skirt around when reason and emotion tell us it just doesn't make sense in our situation.

That leads directly to the third myth about *agape*. *Agape* isn't an emotion; it's a choice. There is a seed of truth here. Love that doesn't act isn't love at all, and all actions start with a choice. We know this intuitively. Scripture confirms it. James chides us: "[If] one of you says to [those in need], 'Go in peace, keep warm, and eat well,' but you don't give them what the body needs, what good is it?"[8] Actions matter, and we certainly have a choice when it comes to loving actions, but it's not too far a jump to thinking actions are all that matter. Then *agape* is only ever an act of the will.

This sounds almost like truth. We choose someone to love, we decide to act in that person's best interests, and we keep our promise. This is often how we see God's love for us. There's a strong implication that this love-of-the-will is far superior, far more elevated, than any old love-of-the-heart. But doesn't the motive matter at all?

Let's take this out of the spiritual realm for a moment. How would this love-of-the-will sound in your life, in your human relationships? Imagine your special someone sitting you down, looking deeply into your eyes, and saying, "Dear one ... precious ... honey ..., I want you to know that I don't love you with some weak emotional love. What I have for you is *agape*. I love you with my will. I have chosen to love you and serve you for your best interests. I've made a promise, and I'm going to keep it. It doesn't really matter that I don't feel any warm emotions toward you."

Would anyone be captivated by this confession? It feels cold, even condescending. Yet because we don't know what to do with the idea of God having emotions, this is exactly what we've made of God's love. *Agape* means God will keep the covenant. That's important, but it's not love.

So tension exists for us as followers of Jesus. How can we be commanded to love if love is an emotion? That doesn't seem fair. How can we love like God when God's love is perfect? That doesn't seem possible. Can we really love our enemies? Can love involve choice, actions, and will, all without devolving into duty?

This brings us to the worst idea of all. The fourth myth? *Agape* is a special kind of love only God has. It's true that God's capacity for *agape* is unique. It encompasses everyone, a love more fierce and strong than we can possibly understand. In the same moment, it can bridge hatred of sin and full sympathy for the people who sin. God's love exists without condition, even including enemies. It can forgive over and over, while maintaining full and fair justice. A love like this is truly beyond us. It seems right, even logical, to suggest that *agape* is something only God has.

Yet this belief becomes a hall pass we use to skip out on actually loving people, especially when it's inconvenient or costly. In pastoral-counseling conversations, I've heard this excuse creep in. "I know God loves him, but I just can't. God can't ask that of me. It's just not fair." We've all seen Christians who disagree profoundly on some controversial issue and treat one another in the most demeaning and disrespectful ways. If you ask them about love, they'll say, "God loves them, but I don't have to like them." Or worse, they'll pull out the old Christian alibi, "We're called to speak the truth in love," as if Scripture somehow frees them from the responsibility to treat others with dignity. *Agape* is something we don't do well, but it's wrong to think for a second it's not supposed to be a part of our lives.

Agape isn't just a theological concept or a philosophical ideal.[9] It's not a contract God has to keep but we don't. *Agape* is real love, really and truly an emotion. It's an emotion God has for you and for the world; it's an emotion you have as well. You may have felt only the edge of what God feels, but you've felt it all the same.

WHAT YOU FEEL WHEN YOU FEEL LIKE GOD

There is an emotional experience all of us have felt, followers of Jesus or not. This emotion connects us most deeply to God's heart. When we feel it, we feel the most like God does. This emotion? Compassion.

Simply, compassion is the feeling you get when you identify with another person such that you are moved to act in that person's best interests. Consider what that means. First, compassion is an emotion. It isn't knowing what's right and doing it. It's a feeling that hits you in your gut.

Second, as an emotion, compassion is unique. It's an emotion of identification. You see someone in a struggle, and something in you goes out to that person. You feel *with* that person. The Latin root of the word combines *com* ("with") and *pati* ("to suffer) to express the idea of suffering with someone.[10] When you feel embarrassment for someone who's blowing her performance onstage or when a friend's pain leaves you in tears, you're bringing into yourself a part of their experience.

This emotion allows you to live up to the apostle Paul's instruction: "Rejoice with those who rejoice; weep with those who weep."[11]

Third, compassion moves you to act. When Lucas was very young, just newly walking, Christina and I would take our kids to a play area at the local mall. Frequent Portland rains leave us with muddy parks, forcing parents to find alternatives. At this particular mall, a long padded couch encloses the play area. In the middle, the kids would climb, run, and play—a scene of lightly controlled chaos. One day a tiny girl stood at the base of the steps to the slide, too scared to climb. Some bigger boys impatiently pushed past her, startling her. She started crying. Lucas watched her for a moment. A sad look spread over his face. Then he toddled over to her and started patting her on the back. He saw her pain. He felt something of what she felt. He went over to be with her, to assure her in his limited way that everything was okay. That's how compassion looks. It moves us to be with people in their experiences.

This is exactly the biblical definition of God's love. John 3 lays out God's love for us:

> God loved the world in this way: He gave His One and Only Son, so that everyone who believes in Him will not perish but have eternal life. For God did not send His Son into the world that He might condemn the world, but that the world might be saved through Him.[12]

God loved the world and saw that we were perishing. This love moved God to act. The Trinity didn't solve our problem in a detached way; God's solution was to enter into our problem to be with us. Theologians call this the incarnation. Through Jesus, God became one of us, the ultimate expression of identification. The King of the universe took on the struggle of human life, the indignity of puberty, the insecurity of poverty, the fear of living in an occupied nation, the injustice of being falsely accused, the dread of being arrested, the physical pain of torture, the heartache of being abandoned, and the suffering of being separated from the Father.

Why did the Father, Son, and Spirit choose this path? Not just to solve our problem. No, God did it to be with us. When Jesus was born, the angel told Mary this baby would be called "Immanuel," a prophetic name meaning "God is with us."[13] God entered into our experience. In Jesus, God identified with us. God felt what we feel. That's compassion.

Don't intellectualize *agape*. It is other-centered love that moves you to identify with another's need and act to help. It's a real emotion you've experienced. When you do, you're feeling in a small way how God feels toward you, toward the people around you, toward the whole world. When you step out to serve someone because of that feeling, you're mirroring God's heart, entering into someone else's experience because of love.

We experience compassion because we're made in God's image and God's heart is compassion. When we feel compassion and act on it, we're living out God's image in the world. In fact, when we feel and act on compassion, we are participating in Jesus' incarnation, furthering the reach of His kingdom in the world.

After I attended the retreat in Minnesota, I imagined sitting down with my own kids in the future, helping them understand their emotions. If that was ever going to be real, I needed to learn their meaning myself.

This vision led me on my path through books, conversations, counseling, journaling, and Bible study, along with frequent references back to the basic emotions chart I kept in my journal. While gathering this knowledge was helpful, there was more to do. Being able to explain the meaning of an emotion is important, but it's a far reach from being able to experience and discern the wisdom each emotion holds.

We've covered the basics of emotions—how they work and where they come from. We've looked specifically at our five most impactful emotions—anger, fear, grief, joy, and love. This information won't be transformative, however, until we begin to practice listening to our emotions. This is where we turn next. How can we use this information to hear wisdom, even God's truth, in our emotions?

QUESTIONS FOR REFLECTION

1. Have you ever considered that *agape* was something you've felt? Or even could feel? Why or why not?

2. The human experience of *agape* is compassion, an emotion of "feeling with" someone else. Can you think of a time you felt with someone else or someone else felt with you? What was that like? How did it affect you?

3. What connection can you see between compassion and Jesus' instruction in Matthew 22:39 to "love your neighbor as yourself"?

Part Four

HOW TO HEAR GOD IN YOUR EMOTIONS

Chapter 16

LEARNING TO PAY ATTENTION

The longest journey is the journey inwards.
Dag Hammarskjöld, *Markings*

Search me, God, and know my heart; test me and
know my anxious thoughts. See if there is any offensive
way in me, and lead me in the way everlasting.
Psalm 139:23–24 NIV

I started riding motorcycles in the summer of 2012. To get your endorsement in Oregon, you must pass a basic rider-training course. I took the course twice and then took the intermediate course before I finally passed the riding test and was legal to ride outside the range. I spent quite a few hours in a classroom learning about equipment, road conditions, and safety. I spent more hours on the range learning how to maneuver under the intimidating eye of experienced trainers.

One morning after riding for a year or more, I was driving my car along the familiar route to my office. As I drove, I noticed each driveway and intersection. I mentally checked in with every other driver, getting a quick sense of where they seemed to be heading. I scanned the road ahead, the next twenty seconds, the next ten seconds. Then I realized what I was doing. Even in my car, I was seeing the road like a biker.

Riding motorcycles safely requires a different mind-set. Your entire world is the next hundred feet of road, encompassing every intersection, every pedestrian, every other vehicle, and the next ten seconds of possibilities. If you want to ride and live, you learn to be profoundly present. I had gotten away with driving my car without this kind of attention for a long time, but on a motorcycle, my survival depends on it. I'd been driving for more than twenty-five years. I thought I was a good driver. I was chagrined to realize I had been driving blind and not even realizing it.

Many of us have been driving blind emotionally for years. We've developed habits and coping mechanisms that work for us, but we've remained emotionally immature and unaware. It took many hours of training and practice on my motorcycle for me to start paying attention in this new way. It will take the same for us to learn how to live with an awareness of our emotions.

A PROCESS FOR UNDERSTANDING YOUR EMOTIONS

Many tools exist to help you recognize and listen to your emotions. There are thoughtful books to get you started, some of which you'll find recommended at www.TheWisdomOfYourHeart.com. Personality inventories and classes can offer insight. Therapists can help you sort through your story. Pastors and spiritual directors can offer guidance in listening for the Holy Spirit's voice. For any of these tools to work, however, you must provide one thing. Without it, you'll be wasting your time.

We're told that experience is the best teacher, but the world is full of people with backpacks jammed full of significant life experiences who are no more mature for them. Maturity doesn't come from having experiences alone but from reflecting on those experiences.

We learn the truth in our emotions by paying attention. Scripture tells us God's word comes to us at times in a "still small voice," with no warning or fanfare.[1] When God speaks through our emotions and the process of unpacking them, it's much like this. Until we learn to pay attention, we'll miss what God might be saying in our intuition and emotional lives. Learning to pay attention is the catalyst for personal, emotional, and spiritual growth.

Paying attention—it sounds so easy. In practice, however, it's one of our most difficult endeavors. A clanging circus of competing voices jars our attention. We're rushed and distracted. We get so much done; our lives require it. But as we dash from crisis to crisis, we don't often stop to listen. Reflecting on and processing our emotions is vital for maturity.

There are many ways to do this, but one rises above all the others: journaling. You may already journal, but I'll wager that if you struggle with understanding your emotions, you haven't been faithful with the practice. This isn't about keeping a diary or writing poetry or sitting in a coffee shop looking reflective. Journaling is a proven method for untangling your thoughts and feelings while uncovering God's guidance.

Journaling is effective precisely because of its limitations. It forces us to slow down. Our culture prefers microwaves to Crock-Pots, but that won't work here. Understanding our own hearts isn't a quick process. Journaling provides focus. Our feelings are often a snarled, multilayered jumble, obscured by unending distraction. The act of writing out our thoughts creates focus we rarely find otherwise. One word at a time, we untangle the knots.

Journaling also enables us to name our experiences. Feelings swirl within, often foggy and unclear. Writing requires the use of particular words. Words create clarity even when we choose the wrong ones. As we see the words written, we can immediately recalibrate. "No, that's not quite right. It's more like this...." Each sentence can be a step closer to clarity.

Finally, journaling gives us a record of our learning. Over time, like a landscape emerging as the morning fog burns off, we begin to see the hidden, unconscious patterns and programs we've been living with.

I'm going to give you a journaling process that will help you exercise the skills of emotional awareness as a part of Christian discipleship. For some of you, these are practices you intuitively understand. You may already even do something similar. Your story and personal wiring have allowed you to live more connected to your emotions. God bless you! But for others like me, this process will be revolutionary. And hard.

After practice, this process can be done mentally, but it's hard work. Until it becomes familiar, it's best to go through the process, step by step, in your journal. The forced focus and reflection of journaling makes the process tangible.

This process is a sequence. It mirrors the natural order of our emotional-response system, bringing it into our awareness. Only there can we reflect, learn, and invite God to teach us. This will lead us to the wisdom within our emotions.

The sequence is recalled with five words—the five As:

> Attend
>
> Articulate
>
> Ask
>
> Assay
>
> Apply

In the beginning, this may seem awkward or artificial. If you're like me, you may find the process takes quite a bit of time. Trust that the more you do it, the more intuitive and easy it will become.

ATTEND: NOTICE YOUR FEELINGS

One of my motorcycle instructors, a twenty-five-year riding veteran, was also a pilot with the Air National Guard. He trained newbie bikers on the weekends and trained fighter pilots during the week. He asked our group what we thought the most crucial riding ability was. We called out our suggestions. Knowing how to lay a bike down safely? Countersteering? The ability to pull off evasive turns? No. More important than any of these, he said, is awareness. If you're aware, you may never need to use those other skills at all. Awareness keeps fighter pilots and motorcycle riders alive. It's just as vital for emotional maturity.

The first step in hearing the truth in our emotions is to pay attention. We attend. This is an old word. It shows up today in the word *attendant* and the idea of an "attending physician." The word meant "to stay or wait with someone, to be present with that person." Picture someone sitting close beside you, compassionately observing what's happening with you. This is what we do for ourselves when we attend.

Our emotional-response system provides us with two kinds of information. First, there is the change in body state and those familiar physiological responses. Second, there is the collection of thoughts accompanying the body state. These are what we watch for.

Early in my emotional recovery, all I could manage was to notice that I was, in fact, feeling something in my body. Not a high bar! My busy, distracted thoughts were of no help. My body, however, would always let me know. Was I feeling flushed? Tense? Was I feeling discomfort in my gut? (That's almost always where emotions show up for me.) Physiological indicators like these all told me the truth: emotions were stirring! At first, that's as far as I could get, but it was a start.

Later on, I began noticing the mind-sets and thoughts that accompanied these bodily changes. These were harder to see. I've worn glasses since the fourth grade, looking at the world through lenses so long, I sometimes forget I'm even wearing them. It's embarrassing to ask my wife whether she's seen my glasses and have her tell me they're on my face! Our mind-sets are much the same. It's hard to see your own mind-set because it's just the way you see the world around you. It takes practice to be able to notice when a certain mind-set is shaping your thinking.

Was I feeling a pull toward something or a push away? Was anxiety pervading my thoughts? Was a mood of frustration shaping my interaction with a person? Was my mind occupied with sad, scary, or disturbing thoughts?

The starting point of understanding your emotions is to attend. Without judgment or the need to explain, you inventory what is apparently true of you. You might even ask the Holy Spirit to help you see accurately. Review the state of your body and mind. In simple, nonjudgmental terms, describe the responses you notice.

- **What is the physiological state of my body right now?** Hot or cold? Relaxed or tense? Are there particular places of tightness or pain? Has the pace of breathing and heartbeat changed? Is there anything new or different in my body state that coincides with the experience of emotion?
- **What is the tone of my thoughts right now?** Busy, slow, distracted, focused? Negative or positive? Pulled toward something or pushing away from something? Is there anything new or different in my mind and thoughts that coincides with the emotional experience?

After taking a scan of your body and mind, you might note something like this:

> Right now my leg is bouncing. I'm tapping my fingers on the desk. My breathing has sped up. My mind is buzzing with a swarm of anxious thoughts.

My shoulders feel heavy, pressed down. My neck is sore. There is a weight on my chest. My thoughts are dark and slow. I'm feeling dread, pressure, and a distinct desire to leave.

You notice and take inventory. There is no story yet. You're not looking for a cause or even trying to name the emotion. Don't rush. This first step is simply the practice of noticing. Instead of reacting or striking out or going into denial, or any of the other habitual reactions you've become comfortable with, stop and take note. What's going on in you?

Sounds like an easy prescription, doesn't it? Pay attention. Yet for some, it's mightily hard. Mental distraction, noise, emotional manipulation, denial, and lack of experience all clutter and obstruct. For a long time, the main way I knew I was feeling strong emotions was because I got agitated or angry. This almost always coincided with a churning gut. I didn't notice this connection until my therapist pointed it out. (I was always blaming the last meal I ate!) "Just sit with it," she said. Simple words, but a difficult and disagreeable practice. Unfortunately, you can't understand what your emotions mean if you don't notice them. You can't deal with them if you don't stop and feel them. So, attend.

ARTICULATE: NAME YOUR EXPERIENCE

Once, Jesus confronted a man possessed by demons. The exchange is fascinating.[2] Jesus asked the demons for their name. There is a long-standing tradition that if you can name an evil spirit, you gain authority over it. We find this to be true in many areas of life. When we can name something, we gain a measure of understanding. This allows us to respond appropriately.

Articulating is about putting a name to what your mind and body are experiencing. If you can't name your feeling, you're liable to just be reactive. On a recent hike, I started feeling a painful pressure when my right foot hit the ground, a pointed irritation. I've had some experience with this kind of pain before, so I could name it. I had a rock in my shoe. Knowing this, I was able to solve the problem. I knew it wasn't the shoe or the trail or some malicious hiker near me. I slipped off my shoe and dumped out the offending rock. Hike saved.

Some of us don't have the emotional experience to name our discomfort. When some emotional irritant causes us pain, we just keep walking and grumbling. Maybe we blame the shoe or the trail or the people around us. It's a silly mental picture, a grumpy hiker hobbling along heaping curses on his boot, the trail, and everything else. Absurd, yes, but this is how many of us deal with our emotions.

How you articulate your feelings will depend on how much experience and personal insight you have. At first, just knowing you're feeling emotions may be hard enough. It took me quite a while to be able to name feelings other than anger. It took practice. I saw a skilled therapist. I journaled pages and pages. I kept going back to my handy basic emotions chart. As time passed, things changed. Instead of emotions washing over me like a sneaker wave, I could feel them and know what I was feeling. If I could do that, I could learn, grow, and maybe even respond appropriately.

Review what you noticed about your body. Those physiological markers always have meaning. A hot, flushed feeling in the face could signal anger, embarrassment, or shame. Hands shaking with adrenaline could mean excitement or rage. A heavy feeling in the gut and tightness in the chest could mean fear. Consider the frame of mind you noticed. Dire thoughts, sad thoughts, blaming thoughts? Noticing these can help you get clear about what you're feeling. As you review what you noticed, give those experiences a name.

Do the bouncing leg, tapping fingers, and buzzing mind seem more like the energy of positive anticipation? Or do they seem more like agitation and anxiety?

Do the heavy pressure and dark thoughts seem more like the ache of regret or more like fear of something in the future?

You're not looking for the cause just yet, although you might have some sense of it. You're not judging the feelings for their accuracy or helpfulness. You're just trying to put a fair name to what you're experiencing.

Get as clear as you can. If you're having a hard time, you can examine the feelings more closely with questions like these:

- **Is this feeling essentially a pull toward something or a push away from something?** Refer back to the basic emotions chart in chapter 10. Each of the emotions is identified as a push or pull emotion. This can narrow down the choices quite a bit.
- **What is this feeling definitely not?** Can you rule out obvious choices you're not feeling? You can

use the basic emotions chart to help you think
through the options.

- **What does this feeling remind you of?** Does
some past experience come to mind with this
feeling? What were you feeling then? How is this
different or similar?

Remember, you can be feeling multiple emotions at the same
time. Ask the Holy Spirit to help you have clarity. If your circumstance is complex, you may need an objective third party to help you
talk it through. In any case, your work is to name your emotional
reality without judgment or censoring. Your emotion isn't good or
bad; it just is. You're not doing anything about it yet, just noticing
and naming.

ASK: CONSIDER THE MEANING

Emotions always tell you the truth, but many times they are telling you a different truth than you first think. In this step, you're
looking for why you're feeling what you're feeling. This can be as
simple as connecting the dots between what you're feeling and the
circumstances you're in. Sometimes the emotion is emerging not
from your immediate circumstances but from your history. In more
complicated situations, you might need counsel from someone who
can see your situation with more objectivity than you can.

The goal is to make a clear connection between what you're feeling and why you're feeling it. Ask, "Why am I feeling these things?"
Expect what comes to mind first not to be the full answer. It might

even be denial or self-delusion. This is a good time to ask the Holy Spirit for discernment.

I recall one particular interaction with a friend that felt off. He expected me to do something for him, something I had previously committed to do. My friend brought this commitment up in conversation. As he did, my gut twisted and I felt threatened. In the past, my response would have been to backpedal or explain why he was wrong or power up and restore my sense of control.

This time, I didn't. Instead, I acknowledged what my friend was saying and then dismissed myself from the conversation. As soon as I could, I pulled out my journal for a basic inventory. I went back to my basic emotions chart to look at what those feelings might mean. (Yes, I kept one of those in my journal for more than a year.) Then I asked myself whether those meanings made sense in my situation. Here's an excerpt from my journal:

> My stomach is all twisty. I'm tense and jumpy. I'm feeling like I need to defend myself. Why? I have a good relationship with this person. He's not out to get me. So what's going on? Well, I feel like I'm in conflict. Why? Did we have a fight? No. I think I feel angry. Why? What does anger generally mean? Anger is the emotion you feel when, in your own private logic, you feel violated. Do I feel violated right now? Yeah, I do. Why? Did he do anything to me? No. Was he asking for something I hadn't promised him? No. So how was I violated? Well, I'm upset he even brought it up. Why is he checking up on me?

As I wrote, I realized I was feeling untrusted. We'd been friends for a long time. If he didn't trust me now, what did that mean for our friendship? As I reflected on these questions, feelings of insecurity surfaced.

I started with the basic meanings of emotions from my basic emotions chart. This allowed me to ask clarifying questions of my own feelings. Because I was still new to this, the process took a while, but by the end, I could say clearly what I was feeling. Then I could sort out which part was reasonable.

Start with what you already have gathered and see where it leads. You might proceed like this:

- **In my body, I'm feeling _____, and in my mind I'm experiencing _____.** You're recounting your observations from the first step—attending.
- **These things may indicate I'm feeling _____.** You're noting the name you've given your feelings in the second step—articulating.
- **The core meaning of this emotion is _____.** Recall the primary meaning of the emotion you're feeling, perhaps referring to the basic emotions chart.
- **Looking at both my outer circumstances and my inner experience, how might this emotion make sense?** If anger is the emotion of being violated, am I being violated right now? If so,

how and by whom? If sadness is the emotion of
loss, what loss am I experiencing?

Asking is about gaining clarity. You ask your emotions for the
data they contain. You ask yourself what might be contributing to
those emotions. You can extend the inquiry by getting the perspective of a trusted friend or counselor. You ask God for discernment to
know what wisdom these emotions are carrying.

ASSAY: WEIGH THE VALUE

Having *attended, articulated,* and *asked,* you now have a fuller and
clearer picture of your emotions. Remember, emotions are neither
right nor wrong. They're information about our inner world and
outer circumstances. Those feelings give us a dashboard warning
light and the energy of motivation. However, the warning light
and the motivation you're feeling can be helpful or unhelpful.
Learning to tell the difference is where we move from information
to wisdom.

Emotionally immature people are often overwhelmed by their
emotions. They may seem reactive and out of control. One young
man I knew became unpredictable and violent when anger struck
him. He destroyed at least four smartphones in the course of three
years, smashing them in fits of anger. He sometimes left holes in
walls or windows. He was always remorseful later but honestly
believed he couldn't control himself when he got mad. His anger
was real. It carried important information about his heart and
circumstances, but he was unable to hear through all his interior

emotional noise. Invariably, his anger alienated people and led to more hurt and more anger.

As we become more emotionally mature, we can sit with our feelings and listen to them without becoming overwhelmed. This allows us access to the tool that can transform our emotional experience: the ability to evaluate what we're feeling.

In the gold-rush days of the American West, a prospector would bring anything he found to the town assayer. The assayer's job was to sort the metals, separating the gold from the iron pyrite, the valuable from the worthless. The assayer would weigh the remaining gold, letting the prospector know its value.

As we mature spiritually and emotionally, we become better equipped to sort out what is emotionally valuable from what is just noise. We can identify the stories emerging in our minds and determine whether those stories are truthful. More importantly, we can decide whether those stories are helpful to us.

When I felt defensive and angry about my friend checking up on me, I had to weigh my emotions. Though it seemed my friend didn't trust me, was this true? I didn't know; it was just my feeling. How much weight should I give my story? My experience over time suggested we had a trusting relationship, so the past didn't line up with my current feeling. That was a clue to look deeper.

So I did. I journaled and prayed over this interaction. As I reflected, a new question surfaced. Was my perceived injury really about our relationship, or was it a manifestation of my need to be seen as credible and in control? Was this really about my pride? Maybe God was nudging me. The more I reflected, the clearer it became. My sense of value has long been constructed from bricks of performance. If this person doubted my ability to come through, that doubt was a threat to my value. When I realized this, I could weigh my emotions more clearly. They were telling me truth, but it wasn't truth about my friend or our relationship. The emotional energy I was feeling came from my own baggage. It wasn't fair to blame my friend for my emotional response. I weighed that interpretation and decided it wasn't gold.

Assaying means weighing the story forming in your mind. You evaluate the interpretation you're making of your emotional response, determining whether it's worth further emotional investment or action. There are several facets of your emotional experience you can evaluate by asking the following questions:

- **In my story, the object of my emotions is _____. Is this interpretation accurate?** The object is what is eliciting the emotion. The person violating you, the thing you lost, the circumstance bringing you joy, and so on. Is this thing really the cause of your emotional response? Often what triggered you is just a flag indicating something deeper.
- **In my story, am I denying any aspect of my own responsibility?** Is any part of your story a way to shift blame onto someone or something else so you can feel better about the situation?
- **Is the level of emotional energy I'm experiencing appropriate given what happened?** Is the intensity of your emotions in proportion to

what you experienced? Are you experiencing too little or too much emotional energy? A disproportionate emotional response almost always indicates something deeper is at stake. Perhaps your circumstances have triggered something from your own past.

- **The emotion I'm experiencing is moving me to _____. Will this response be helpful or hurtful?** Does the action you're moved to take align with who you want to be or with who you believe God is asking you to be?

In passing I've mentioned a few times the role God plays in this process for a follower of Jesus. I've suggested asking the Holy Spirit for discernment or asking God to lead. But let me be abundantly clear, in case that wasn't sufficient: our emotional and spiritual lives intertwine. As we become aware of the emotional response we're experiencing and the story emerging from it, we bring all of this to God and invite God to give us clarity and understanding. We are not alone as we listen to and unpack our emotions; the Holy Spirit is with us. We can use this process to have a higher level of personal insight about our emotions, but if we walk these steps inviting the Holy Spirit to guide, they can become transformational.

Questions like these may be fruitful for bringing your emotions before God:

- **Do my emotions on this issue align with God's emotions as I understand them?** For example, if you're angry, is it something God would also be angry about? Or are you being selfishly angry?

- **Is God surfacing something in my character or personal story that needs attention?** For example, maybe you're noticing that a particular struggle is coming up over and over again. Maybe God is inviting you to look at that area.

- **Is my pain or reactivity truly from some kind of violation I've experienced, or is it because of injured pride?** Is some idol you've held close screaming to reassert control?

- **Does this emotional response reveal woundedness or sin in my heart? Does it reveal spiritual growth?** For example, was your emotional energy disproportionate, showing that you're nursing a wound? Or are you emotionally triggered by something less quickly, showing that you've grown or experienced healing?

- **Do the actions I'm feeling moved to take reflect Jesus' character?** How might you respond in a way that expresses emotional integrity but is also loving?

APPLY: ACT WITH INTENTION

Having evaluated your emotional response and the story emerging from it, what will you do?

Knowing what you now know, you have new freedom. You're no longer bound to the same old reactions, driven by a passing feeling or the unconscious pressure of your own story. Now you can make an intentional choice.

Emotions exist to move us. The energy building within us during an emotional response dissipates only when we take action. That's why we react. The goal of emotional maturity, however, is to channel this emotional energy into constructive and life-giving actions. Emotional discipleship is the process of learning how to channel this energy into a life that reflects and honors Christ.

In my experience with the friend I felt was checking up on me, there were several actions I could take. As I assayed the situation, I could see this wasn't really about my friend at all. I didn't need to nurse anger toward him. I didn't even need to talk with him about it, necessarily. Instead, I needed to address my internal fears. I confessed my pride to God. I acknowledged, once again, that I keep finding my value in performance rather than in my identity in Christ. The next time I interacted with this person, I noticed I was able to be in the moment, not caught up at all in worrying about his judgment of me. I was excited, since it doesn't always go this well.

The appropriate response for you will vary depending on the situation. Do you need to have a conversation? Do you need to take responsibility? Has a deeper issue been uncovered that needs prayer or counseling? Is God leading you to act in some way? To give, to serve, to sit with, to advocate for, to stand up for someone?

As you choose, you channel the emotional energy you're feeling into action. Instead of reacting or exploding or stuffing your feelings, you have listened and learned, and now you're free to move forward in a healthy way.

THE FIVE As: LISTENING TO FIND WISDOM

This process weaves together the pursuits of knowing ourselves and knowing God. We aren't led by emotions or living by rote dogma. We aren't ignoring the Spirit's guidance. We bring who we are to God, surrendering our whole selves—including our emotions— to God. This is the essence of growing in Christ. Pete Scazzero summarizes this point perfectly: "At the very least, the call of discipleship includes experiencing our feelings, reflecting on our feelings, and then thoughtfully responding to our feelings under the lordship of Jesus."[3]

We *attend*, noticing what is happening in our bodies and minds. We *articulate*, naming our experience so we can better understand and deal with it. We *ask*, searching our emotions and circumstances and seeking God's guidance to better understand the message being delivered. We *assay*, weighing the story emerging in our minds so we can discern what is worthwhile and what is not. We *apply*, acting with intention so every emotional response can find its expression in life-giving, loving actions. With practice, we grow in our experience and ease with this process. This is what it means to mature emotionally.

QUESTIONS FOR REFLECTION

1. Do you presently journal? What is your journaling process like? If you don't journal, why not?

2. Do you have some kind of practice for reflecting on and working through your emotions? If so, what is that process like? Which part of the five As is missing? If you don't have a process, why not? How might a process like this be helpful to you?

3. Consider Pete Scazzero's quotation at the end of this chapter. How are you going to incorporate this kind of process into your life?

Chapter 17

WE GROW WELL WHEN WE FEEL WELL

I will give you a new heart and put a new spirit within you; I
will remove your heart of stone and give you a heart of flesh.
Ezekiel 36:26

When Jesus saw [the invalid] lying there and knew he had already
been there a long time, He said to him, "Do you want to get well?"
John 5:6

For our tenth wedding anniversary, Christina and I took a cruise. We departed from San Juan, Puerto Rico, lazily circling the Caribbean for seven sun-soaked days. Most of the other passengers were Puerto Rican. Turns out Puerto Ricans who want to take a vacation can't drive to Disneyland! The ship was filled with vibrant, enthusiastic Latin energy.

Christina wanted me to take dance lessons with her. Of course, the dance lessons on board were all Latin dances—salsa, rumba, and merengue. This wasn't the American prom shuffle! Surrounded by

Puerto Ricans who had been dancing since they could walk, I was self-conscious and intimidated. The merengue was the easiest to learn, we were told, so that's where we started. Quite a distance from the community I grew up in, where dancing was forbidden!

I've never really enjoyed watching people dance, but I did on that cruise. Even the elderly Puerto Rican couples who shuffled along the deck would transform into stylish dancers when the music started. I had to count steps in my head. They just danced, grace in motion.

Of course, it's not only Puerto Ricans who love to dance. Every child everywhere dances. Play the music, and they start to bounce. Even buttoned-up stiffs will toe-tap or head-bop to the right music. Insecurity and cultural pressure squeeze the dance out of us as we get older. That is unless we live in a culture that values and teaches dance. Even the awkward Puerto Rican teenagers became fluent dancers when the band started. They grew up with dance being modeled, valued, and taught.

Emotional maturity is much the same. For most of us, our emotional-response systems work right out of the box, but many of us have lived in cultures—families, churches, communities—where the emotional dance wasn't modeled, valued, or taught. Now, as adults, many of us aren't even aware of everything we're missing.

LEARNING TO DANCE

This summer Christina and I took our kids to the Saint Helens Fourth of July celebration. Saint Helens is a small Oregon town on the banks of the Columbia River, about thirty miles north of Portland. It was just the right speed for our eight- and ten-year-olds.

They rode ponies, got their faces painted, and even got to honk the air horns on the municipal roadwork trucks. I guess that's an attraction in small towns. We ate a fresh blueberry pie. Not slices—half an unsliced pie in a take-out box. With plastic spoons. Before the fireworks, a live band played high-energy radio hits.

As the band played, my family and I pressed through the crowd until we were close to the stage. We danced and sang at the top of our voices. My son bopped up and down to the beat with a big grin. My daughter, all whirling arms and tangled hair, danced as if she were the only one in the crowd.

I glanced at the amphitheater seats along the edge of the crowd behind us and smiled. In another part of my life, I would have been sitting back there, enjoying the music at a safe distance, missing out and not even knowing it. Too self-conscious and afraid, I was unwilling to look silly.

Those merengue lessons on our anniversary cruise were the first time I had ever really danced. On purpose. Where people could see. That was six years before, just about the time crisis and depression forced me onto this path of emotional healing. Getting comfortable dancing in front of other people has taken a long time. It's been awkward and scary, but it's opened up a new experience of joy for me.

Getting comfortable facing and listening to my emotions has taken a long time too. It's a continuing journey. I still journal. I still find myself needing to walk through the five As when unexpected emotions overtake me. If I don't spend intentional time with others who can speak truth to me, I fall back into old habits. I have to pay close attention so that the stories I'm constructing in my mind don't keep me from seeing what's true.

I'm still the same person, the firstborn, adopted son of a conservative pastor's family who wrestles with performance and people pleasing. I am, however, less likely to overreact. I'm able to listen to others in a way I never could have before, and I'm much quicker to apologize and own my responsibility. I can be present with people, even with myself. I'm softer. Some days I'm even happy! Clearly I have further to go, but as with those penciled height markings on a kitchen doorframe, I can see evidence that I'm growing up.

Learning to listen to my emotions has opened up spiritual growth for me in a way I haven't experienced since I was young. My sense of God is deeper and more present. My faith has shifted toward trust in a person rather than certainty based on my doctrine and holiness. Even my more conventional faith practices—like reflecting on Scripture, praying, and gathering for worship—are infused with a depth that had for years seemed lost to me.

Pete Scazzero wrote:

> To feel is to be human. To minimize or deny what we feel is a distortion of what it means to be image bearers of our personal God. To the degree that we are unable to express our emotions, we remain impaired in our ability to love God, others, and ourselves well.[1]

Impaired in our ability to love. That was my experience. For years I wasn't feeling well. I don't mean I was sick. I mean I wasn't doing the feeling part of life well. I wasn't paying attention. I was ignoring the flashing dashboard lights. That cost me and those I love dearly. But God's gracious gift of pain, as well as the timely help of good friends and a skilled counselor, taught me what I had never understood before. Emotions aren't a flaw in God's plan. They aren't a sinful failure of God's perfect design. They're an integral part of our being, designed to tell us the truth and move us. Perhaps this is nothing new for you, but for me, it was a revolution.

TURNING TOWARD A VIBRANT REALITY

We read in Ephesians 4:11–13 that God's purpose in our lives is to grow us up in the image of Christ. This includes the whole of who we are. Emotional maturity contributes to healthy relationships. That's obvious. Less obvious is that this extends to our relationship with God as well. You can't have intimacy if you can't feel. Without intimacy, your relationships stay shallow and transactional. Unfortunately, that's a fair description of the relationship so many have with God. Shallow and transactional. Reading more Scripture, praying more, serving the poor, and giving more tithes won't deepen that relationship. Depth comes with intimacy, and without an emotional connection, intimacy is impossible.

Deuteronomy 4:29 says that when you seek God "with all your heart and all your soul," you will find God. This isn't talking about a propositional, doctrinal faith, as essential as good doctrine may be. This is calling us to a fervency of heart. We were made to engage God with all of who we are—heart, soul, mind, and strength, and relationships as well. Isn't this the kind of fully engaged life we see in the apostles and the early church? Isn't that what inspires us about them? They didn't go to the stake, the lions, and the sword because it was just the right thing to do. The heroes of our faith, who took risks, challenged the status quo, started hospitals, fought slavery, opened soup kitchens and orphanages, or took care of lepers in the streets—these heroes weren't doing these things only because of duty. For some, compassion led them to feel the needs of the people around them. For others, anger empowered them to see and stand against injustice. A profound love for God moved them to set aside personal security in the face of real danger. They lived this way because they were moved. So why not us?

The modern church in many places is dry and brittle. We need the Holy Spirit to move, but can we hear the Spirit if we're unable to sit still and be quiet? The voice of the Spirit is most often still and small, discernible only in our hearts' quiet depths. Without the ability to listen to our emotions and discern wisdom there, we risk naming our own preferences and fears as the Holy Spirit's leading. Sidelining and second-classing our emotions has led us to this place. We need authentic emotional maturity in the lives of individual followers of Jesus, nurtured in communities that include emotional wholeness in their ongoing process of discipleship. Anything less is to deny that God created us as integrated beings, and it invites people into a hobbled spirituality that can never speak to their whole lives.

Consider these words from authors Dan Allender and Tremper Longman: "Emotions are the language of the soul. They are the cry that gives the heart a voice."[2] Our churches need to hear the voice of the heart. Again, Pete Scazzero: "Christian spirituality, without an integration of emotional health, can be deadly—to yourself, your relationship with God, and the people around you."[3] For our emotional health, for our relationships, for our spiritual vitality, we must hear the voice of our hearts.

Maybe you're a more emotionally connected person than I was. You've listened to my story with an eyebrow raised, wondering how someone could be so unaware. For you, I suspect, the challenge of discipling your emotional life is to bring it under God's guidance. Hearing when God speaks in your emotions isn't as simple as just doing whatever you feel. You may be comfortable being an emotional person, but are you ready to let God shape your emotions?

Or perhaps you were nodding your head as I shared my journey. Maybe the idea of bringing emotion into your life of faith sounds scary, out of control, even in conflict with your theology. For you, the challenge of discipling your emotional life may be to let go of your need to be in control all the time. Consider the possibility that ignoring, denying, or repressing your emotions shuts you off from an important avenue of God's guidance. Perhaps God is inviting you to leave what's comfortable behind so you can heal and grow.

"Today," the psalmist wrote, "if you hear His voice: Do not harden your hearts."[4] A hard and stubborn heart can keep us from acting on God's direction, but worse, a hard heart can keep us from hearing God at all. While it's not accurate to say that the hard heart in Scripture is entirely about emotions, it's fair to say that emotional immaturity is an ingredient. My emotional immaturity and brokenness made it very hard for me to hear others and hard to separate God's guidance from my own wishes and fears.

Emotional numbness, denial, and self-justification can become a scaly armor, but under God's caring hand, the hardness of sin, pride, trauma, and fear can soften. Then we'll find ourselves able to feel. Perhaps you've given up hope that a change like this is possible. I had. I had tried so many times to change myself, and nothing I did made a lasting difference. But we aren't left alone in this. God promises aid: "I will give you a new heart and put a new spirit within you; I will remove your heart of stone and give you a heart of flesh."[5] This is what growing spiritually often looks like. We transition, often slowly and painfully, from a hard heart to a soft one.

The process is painful. It must be. Part of the reason we've avoided our emotions is because there is pain to feel. Feeling that pain is a good and healing part of coming to life. That's what this journey really is—coming back to life. The abundant life means living fully as the people God made us to be, maturing in the image of Jesus. That includes all of us, every part. This is a kind of conversion—not the conversion of faith when we choose to follow Jesus but the long conversion, like a seed becoming a vibrant plant bearing beautiful fruit. We try and fail, and by grace we try again. We learn to listen, letting go of self-justifying stories. In doing so, we discover that the Teacher of our souls isn't dead words on a page but an active, living Spirit calling us forward.

We're called away from being self-centered spiritual and emotional infants, demanding with tears and temper that the world keep us safe and meet our every need. We're called toward spiritual and emotional adulthood, where we love others as ourselves and we're authentically growing in "love, joy, peace, patience, kindness, goodness, faith, gentleness, [and] self-control."[6]

Unless your discipleship includes emotion, this change of heart surely won't happen. Spirituality without emotions isn't full or healthy. But there is something better: emotional maturity enables us to live with soft hearts that are able to listen and feel, that come to beat in time with God's own heart, moving us to act in ways that embody God's love. No longer will unnecessary fear bind us; no longer will self-justifying and self-protective anger drive us. We'll be able to truly grieve our losses and release them without bitterness. And we'll be able to feel deep joy, wonder, and happiness. This is the gift God gave us with emotions: a life richly experienced and understood, with wisdom from the heart, available for all.

QUESTIONS FOR REFLECTION

1. Did you grow up in an environment where emotional maturity was valued, modeled, and taught? How did your experience shape you? How do you want your life to be different in this regard?

2. How will authentic emotional maturity in the lives of individual Christians shape the churches they're a part of? How could it change the culture of Christianity? How might it change the experience the world has of Christians?

3. What have you learned over the course of this book that you want to apply to your life today? How will you take that from a good intention into real action?

NEXT STEPS AND USEFUL RESOURCES

Well, you've made it! Thank you so much for the attention and time you've given to this material. It is my deepest hope that what you've read here will encourage and equip you for a healthier, more vibrant life and relationship with God.

The process of growth can start with a book, but it takes investment and intentionality to continue. I hope I can support you in your growth beyond the pages of this book. To that end, I've assembled a variety of additional resources and tools to help you work through the material. Find these resources at www.TheWisdomOfYourHeart.com, including

- recommended books to help you go deeper on the book topics, including anger, grief, loss, identity in Christ, and many others;
- links to blogs and other relevant online resources, such as how to find a good therapist, how to support someone who is grieving, and more; and

- downloadable and printable resources that support the content of each chapter, including a specially formatted basic emotions chart you can print out and keep handy for your personal use.

Often our best learning happens when we can dialogue with others. At www.TheWisdomOfYourHeart.com, you'll also find a series of video courses to help you more deeply engage the content of this book. These courses have been designed for small groups, but individuals will find them valuable as well. Here is what the courses include:

- **Course 1: "The Wisdom of Your Heart."** This six-week course is offered free to any individual or small group. Meant to accompany the book, this course walks through the six major book themes. Each week includes a short video introduction, a reading assignment from the book, discussion questions, and a journaling assignment.
- **Course 2: "Uncovering the Story That Shapes Your Emotions."** This six-week course expands on the idea of our personal stories, introduced in chapter 2 of the book, and walks through a process of identifying the story and inherited maps that affect our emotional lives.
- **Course 3: "Under the Hood of Your Emotions."** This six-week course expands on chapters 8–15 in the book, looking at the inner workings of our

emotional-response system and the meaning of different emotions. This course is ideal for people who need additional coaching as they grow in understanding their own emotions.

- **Course 4: "Learning to Listen to Emotion's Truth."** This six-week course presents a step-by-step walk-through of the five As, the listening process taught in chapter 16, for people who would like to learn how to use this process in their daily lives.

NOTES

PREFACE

1. Pete Scazzero has been deeply influential in my journey of healing and emotional recovery. I recommend all his books to you. You'll hear from him a number of times in these pages. He is the founding pastor of New Life Fellowship Church in Queens, New York. He and his wife, Geri, have spent nearly two decades working to understand the role of emotions in the life of a church and to create practical ways to help Christians mature emotionally.

2. Peter Scazzero, *Emotionally Healthy Spirituality: Unleash a Revolution in Your Life in Christ* (Nashville: Thomas Nelson, 2006), 17.

CHAPTER 1

1. See summary in Jonaki Bose et al., *Key Substance Use and Mental Health Indicators in the United States: Results from the 2015 National Survey on Drug Use and Health*, pub. SMA 16-4984, NSDUH series H-51 (Rockville, MD: Center for Behavioral Health and Statistics Quality, 2016), www.samhsa.gov/data /sites/default/files/NSDUH-FFR1-2015/NSDUH-FFR1-2015/NSDUH -FFR1-2015.htm.

2. Cindy Brosh, my former therapist and a beta reader of this manuscript, pointed out that our experience of this comparison also includes a great number of embedded gender assumptions. Being called emotional in our culture often carries feminine associations. A man who is called emotional is labeled with language that has often been used to describe women. His level of comfort with his own feminine side will influence the level of discomfort he feels with the label. Being called reasonable in our culture also carries an equivalent

masculine tone. Stereotypically, men are supposed to be reasonable, and women are supposed to be emotional.

3. Plato's description of the horses shows his bias against emotion. He wrote, "First the charioteer of the human soul drives a pair, and secondly one of the horses is noble and of noble breed, but the other quite the opposite in breed and character. Therefore in our case the driving is necessarily difficult and troublesome." See Plato, *Plato in Twelve Volumes*, trans. Harold N. Fowler, vol. 9, *Phaedrus*, (Cambridge: Harvard University Press, 1925), sec. 246b, www.perseus.tufts.edu/hopper/text?doc=Perseus%3Atext%3A1999.01.0174%3Atext%3DPhaedrus%3Asection%3D246b. For an accessible explanation that goes further into Plato's teaching on this subject, see *Wikipedia*, s.v. "Chariot Allegory," last modified January 18, 2017, http://en.wikipedia.org/wiki/Chariot_Allegory.

4. For a quick and easy summary of the Stoics' teachings, as well as some of the more notable figures in that movement, see *Wikipedia*, s.v. "Zeno of Citium," last modified April 1, 2017, http://en.wikipedia.org/wiki/Zeno_of_Citium; and *Wikipedia*, s.v. "Stoicism," last modified May 3, 2017, http://en.wikipedia.org/wiki/Stoicism.

5. Matthew Elliott, *Feel: The Power of Listening to Your Heart* (Carol Stream, IL: Tyndale, 2008), 2.

6. Peter Scazzero, *Emotionally Healthy Spirituality: Unleash a Revolution in Your Life in Christ* (Nashville: Thomas Nelson, 2006), 26.

CHAPTER 2

1. This concept is discussed compellingly in Bessel A. van der Kolk's book *The Body Keeps the Score: Brain, Mind, and Body in the Healing of Trauma* (New York: Viking, 2014).

CHAPTER 3

1. This flaw was covered widely in the news media at the time. Here's one example: Nilay Patel and Adi Robertson, "Wrong Turn: Apple's Buggy iOS 6 Maps Lead to Widespread Complaints," *Verge*, September 20, 2012, www.theverge.com/2012/9/20/3363914/wrong-turn-apple-ios-6-maps-phone-5-buggy-complaints.

2. Another example of the flawed map data affecting people: Brad Reed, "Apple's iOS Maps Pushes Woman to Brink of Madness," *BGR*, February 28, 2014, http://bgr.com/2014/02/28/worst-apple-maps-mistakes/.

3. A potentially dangerous flaw! See Dave Smith, "Apple Maps Fails Again: Alaska Drivers Directed onto Airport Taxiway, No Fix in Sight," *International Business Times*, September 25, 2013, www.ibtimes.com/apple-maps-fails-again-alaska -drivers-directed-airport-taxiway-no-fix-sight-1410830.

4. Very dangerous! See Steven Musil, "Australia Police Discourage Use of Apple Maps App after Rescues," *CNET*, December 9, 2012, www.cnet.com/news /australia-police-discourage-use-of-apple-maps-app-after-rescues/.

5. Romans 1:25.

6. Today we use the word *heart* to refer to the seat of our emotions, but this isn't really what the word meant in its original context. "Heart" in Jeremiah 17:9 is translated from the Hebrew word *leb*. In the Hebrew worldview this referred to the "inner man" and was thought of as the seat of will, conscience, and morality. It was where one "purposed" to do something. Sometimes the word was used to refer to our inner thoughts, or where those thoughts come from. The point of this passage is not that the heart (in our modern usage, relating to emotions) can't be trusted but that *we*, as human beings, are fallen and deceitful.

7. One of several scriptures that address this is Malachi 3:6.

8. James 1:13.

9. James Rowe, "I Would Be like Jesus" © 1911 public domain.

10. Clint Brown, "I Wanna Be More like You" © 1989 Hosanna! Music.

CHAPTER 4

1. Luke 10:25, 27.

2. Jesus was quoting the Shema, the central prayer of Judaism that includes Deuteronomy 6:4–5. The idea that we are whole and integrated beings runs the length of Scripture, because it is God's design for us.

3. Arguments abound regarding how the early chapters of Genesis should be read and interpreted. Some view this story as a literal description of events that took place on a certain day in history, sort of divine journalism. Others think it's a metaphorical story or even mythology. These arguments often obscure something important that remains true regardless of which side of the debate you favor. Genesis talks about the essential nature of humanity. The biblical view of human nature starts here. We were created in God's image with great care for a good purpose, and we were created as whole beings. The particular mechanism of creation and the various theories of inspiration are far less vital

than we often think, and the heart of the story is far more important than we often acknowledge.

4. I use the older King James Version translation here because it retains the phrase *living soul*, while most modern translations use the phrase *living being*. The newer translations offer a more accurate reading of the Hebrew word *nephesh*—which means "a person, a living being, a creature that breathes, a self"—but the King James translation has so profoundly shaped our spiritual imaginations, it seemed right to use it.

5. Psalm 18:30; Matthew 5:48.

6. Malachi 3:6; James 1:17.

7. Ephesians 4:11–13.

8. "Wait!" you say. "Isn't the purpose of the church evangelism? That's what the Great Commission says in Matthew 28, right?" Yes. But why? Why does evangelism matter? That's what Ephesians 4 is telling us. God wants people saved so they can mature in the image of Christ, now and in eternity. God's endgame for each of us isn't just salvation. It's maturity.

9. Genesis 1:27.

CHAPTER 5

1. My friend Donny reminded me that Curt Cloninger wrote this "God-Views" sketch. An excerpt of it (that unfortunately does not include the box character) can be seen on YouTube at www.youtube.com/watch?v=TWnCB_X0uuM.

2. Colossians 1:15.

3. John 14:9.

4. Matthew 23:27.

5. Mark 10:17–22.

6. Matthew 9:36; 14:14; 15:32; Mark 6:34; 8:2.

7. Matthew 20:34; Mark 1:41; 9:22.

8. Luke 7:13–15.

9. See, for example, the New American Standard Bible (NASB).

10. Matthew 8:27.

11. Matthew 9:8 is one example.

12. Matthew 22:22 is one example.

13. Matthew 27:14.

14. Luke 19:41.

15. John 11:32–35.

16. Mark 14:34.

17. As a child, I was taught that Jesus was punishing the people who were making
    noise in the temple, so we should always be quiet and prayerful in the sanctu-
    ary. Of course, it makes no sense at all that Jesus would create a scene like this
    if He was just advocating for decorum in church.

18. John 2:17.

19. Mark 10:14.

20. John 14:9.

21. Hebrews 1:3 NIV.

22. Colossians 1:15.

23. First Peter 2:22.

CHAPTER 6

1. Trinitarian theology notwithstanding.

2. Genesis 1:25, 31.

3. First Kings 3:10.

4. Matthew 3:17 NIV.

5. Zephaniah 3:17.

6. Jeremiah 31:3 NIV.

7. Genesis 19:19.

8. Genesis 39:21.

9. Exodus 15:13.

10. Numbers 14:18 is just one example of about twenty found throughout the Old
    Testament.

11. Sally Lloyd-Jones, *The Jesus Storybook Bible: Every Story Whispers His Name*
    (Grand Rapids: Zonderkidz, 2007), 36. This phrase is, in my mind, the most
    theologically accurate description of both *agape* and *hesed*. Most children's
    Bibles are theological party favors with the literary quality of a fortune
    cookie. Lloyd-Jones managed to write a children's Bible that is both beautiful
    to read and profound in its theological focus. I have repeatedly used this
    Bible with adults who are new Christians, as it helps solidify in their minds

the overarching narrative of Scripture, with a spotlight on Jesus throughout. Lloyd-Jones' words and Jago's illustrations have made this a true work of art. I cannot recommend it to you enough.

12. Genesis 6:6.

13. Ephesians 4:30.

14. Matthew 19:22.

15. Matthew 26:37.

16. Both Psalm 78:40 and Isaiah 63:10 use the same Hebrew word found in Genesis 6:6, pointing out the many times in the wilderness wanderings that the Israelites' choices caused God sorrow.

17. Deuteronomy 1:34–37.

18. A few examples are Numbers 32:13; 2 Kings 13:3; Job 4:9; Isaiah 13:5; Lamentations 2:2; and Ezekiel 7:8.

19. Isaiah 30:30.

20. Exodus 20:5; Deuteronomy 5:9.

21. Proverbs 6:16–19.

22. Amos 5:21; see also Isaiah 58. "Why is our worship not working?" Israel asked. At length, God responded. Proper religious behavior is meaningless unless it is backed up with care for the needy, the hungry, and the oppressed.

CHAPTER 7

1. "Because I, Yahweh, have not changed, you descendants of Jacob have not been destroyed."

2. "God is not a man who lies, or a son of man who changes His mind."

3. "Every generous act and every perfect gift is from above, coming down from the Father of lights; with Him there is no variation or shadow cast by turning."

4. Genesis 18:16–33.

5. Exodus 32:9–14.

6. Open theism and process theology are current theological conversations discussing the possibility that, in some manner or other, God is experiencing life along with us. Perhaps God doesn't see a specific outcome ahead of time but instead sees all possible outcomes simultaneously. These discussions are controversial in many circles, but we don't have to get mired in those deep

weeds to admit honestly that Scripture suggests that our responses affect God in some real and meaningful way.

7. These three sentences may raise a lot of issues for you. Later in this book, we'll be looking at each of these emotions individually and talking about their meaning, how they show up in the Bible, and how God might use them to communicate with us. So hold on.

8. Acknowledging anthropomorphism is one of the dividing lines between primitive and modern religion. In fact, this line is embedded in the definition of the word. Dictionary.com defines *anthropomorphic* this way: "Ascribing human form or attributes to a being or thing not human, especially to a deity." Modern religion understands when we're talking about spirit; we have only human words to describe it.

9. Among those who accept the omnis, there are a number of differences in interpretation. For example, if God is omniscient, does that mean God knows all the knowledge there is, or does it mean that God knows all knowable knowledge? If God knows only all knowable knowledge, are there domains outside God's knowledge as a matter of nature, or does God self-limit divine knowledge in some way? Perhaps to protect our free will? Clearly, the water gets murky quickly.

CHAPTER 8

1. Antonio R. Damasio, "A Modern Phineas Gage," chap. 3 in *Descartes' Error: Emotion, Reason, and the Human Brain* (New York: Avon Books, 1994).

2. A variety of recent studies have largely discredited the left-brain, right-brain explanation of personality. Even so, it remains a common popular explanation of the differences between people. For more information, see Christopher Wanjek, "Left Brain vs. Right: It's a Myth, Research Finds," *Live Science*, September 3, 2013, www.livescience.com/39373-left-brain-right-brain-myth.html. See also Jared A. Nielsen et al., "An Evaluation of the Left-Brain vs. Right-Brain Hypothesis with Resting State Functional Connectivity Magnetic Resonance Imaging," *PLOS ONE* 8, no. 8 (August 2013): 1–11, http://journals.plos.org /plosone/article?id=10.1371/journal.pone.0071275.

3. A short segment of David Brooks' interview with Dr. Damasio (Aspen Ideas Festival, Aspen, Colorado, July 4, 2009) on his interaction with Elliot can be viewed on YouTube at www.youtube.com/watch?v=1wup_K2WN0I. The full interview is available at Antonio Damasio, "This Time with Feeling," FORA.tv, July 4, 2009, http://fora.tv/2009/07/04/Antonio_Damasio_This_Time _With_Feeling.

4. *Online Etymology Dictionary*, s.v. "emotion," accessed May 16, 2017, www.etymonline.com/index.php?term=emotion.

5. Romans 6:17–18.

6. Matthew 6:33 is one example.

7. Matthew Elliott, *Feel: The Power of Listening to Your Heart* (Carol Stream, IL: Tyndale, 2008), 4.

8. Read the full Gethsemane account in Matthew 26:36–46; Luke 22:39–46; and Mark 14:32–42.

9. Matthew 26:39.

10. Hebrews 12:2.

CHAPTER 9

1. Elizabeth Johnston and Leah Olson, *The Feeling Brain: The Biology and Psychology of Emotions* (New York: W. W. Norton, 2015), 308–9.

2. We share this push-or-pull dynamic with even the simplest of organisms. Every creature needs a certain environment to survive. That ideal environment provides the right food, temperature, shelter, and other necessities for life. The organism will naturally be drawn to these beneficial things. Introduce something destructive into the environment, and the organism will naturally withdraw. A single-celled organism will pull away when the tip of a needle begins to pierce its membrane.

CHAPTER 10

1. Summary of discussion in Antonio Damasio, "Of Appetites and Emotions," chap. 2 in *Looking for Spinoza: Joy, Sorrow, and the Feeling Brain* (Orlando: Harcourt, 2003).

2. Dr. Damasio says: "Feeling, in the pure and narrow sense of the word, was the idea of the body being in a certain way" (Damasio, *Looking for Spinoza*, 85). Feelings are the thought of emotion.

3. For more information, see *Wikipedia*, s.v. "*Lie to Me*," last modified May 15, 2017, https://en.wikipedia.org/wiki/Lie_to_Me.

4. Paul Ekman, "Facial Expressions of Emotion: New Findings, New Questions," *Psychological Science* 3, no. 1 (January 1992): 34–38, www.jstor.org/stable/10 .2307/40062750?ref=search-gateway:1243644dc8df7deca309475a127b73d4.

5. This fascinating experiment was replicated not only multiple times but also in another culture. This suggests that the essential body postures of emotion are hardwired into us and aren't something we learn through imitation or enculturation.

6. Paul J. Whalen et al., "Masked Presentations of Emotional Facial Expressions Modulate Amygdala Activity without Explicit Knowledge," *Journal of Neuroscience* 18, no. 1 (January 1998): 411–18, http://citeseerx.ist.psu.edu /viewdoc/download?doi=10.1.1.336.5325&rep=rep1&type=pdf.

7. Your body state may be different. While many physiological responses are the same from person to person, it also seems to be the case that their order and how conscious we are of them differ. One person may be very aware of a flushed, hot face, while someone else may be aware of a pounding heart. Generally, though, your individual responses will be fairly predictable. For me, learning to identify these physiological responses was the starting point for identifying my emotions.

8. There is a difference between an emotion and a mood. A mood is an ongoing emotional state. For it to continue, it must be fed. This is where we have the capacity to change or continue our emotions, and it's where our moral choice enters in.

9. See Robert Plutchik, "A Structural Model of the Emotions," chap. 8 in *The Emotions*, rev. ed. (Lanham, MD: University Press of America, 1991). Dr. Plutchik was a psychologist, researcher, and college professor. He believed that emotions are the result of natural selection, with each emotion filling a necessary role in survival. Regardless of your beliefs on the origin of humanity, however, Plutchik's insights on the meaning of emotions are insightful and practical. He intuited that each emotion has a specific function in our lives. Essentially, each different emotion is a different warning light on the dashboard of our inner lives. These different indicators have the role of moving us to act in different ways.

10. Plutchik, "Structural Model," 111.

11. Robert Plutchik, *The Emotions*, rev. ed. (Lanham, MD: University Press of America, 1991), 109.

CHAPTER 11

1. In *Emotional Intelligence*, Daniel Goleman summarizes the research of Joseph LeDoux, explaining the role of the amygdala and how easily it short-circuits our brain processes. He writes, "LeDoux's work revealed how the architecture of the brain gives the amygdala a privileged position as an emotional

sentinel.... Sensory signals from eye or ear travel first in the brain to the thalamus, and then—across a single synapse—to the amygdala; a second signal from the thalamus is routed to the neocortex—the thinking brain. This branching allows the amygdala to begin to respond *before* the neocortex." Daniel Goleman, *Emotional Intelligence: Why It Can Matter More Than IQ; and Working with Emotional Intelligence* (London: Bloomsbury, 2004), 17.

2. Robert Solomon, a philosopher and one of the most important emotional theorists, defined it like this: "Anger is basically a judgment that one has been wronged or offended." It's bigger than that, but that's the core. Robert C. Solomon, *True to Our Feelings: What Our Emotions Are Really Telling Us* (New York: Oxford University Press, 2007), 18.

3. Jerry Holt, the counselor who facilitated the retreat on pastoral burnout I attended, introduced this concept to me. The asterisk appended to the definition of *anger* applies to all emotions, not just anger. Our perception of our circumstances is sufficient to cause an emotional response, and our perception isn't always accurate.

4. Galatians 5:19–21: "The works of the flesh are obvious: sexual immorality, moral impurity, promiscuity, idolatry, sorcery, hatreds, strife, jealousy, outbursts of anger, selfish ambitions, dissensions, factions, envy, drunkenness, carousing, and anything similar. I tell you about these things in advance—as I told you before—that those who practice such things will not inherit the kingdom of God."

5. Proverbs 29:11.

6. James 1:19–20.

7. Mark 3:1–5.

8. See Galatians 3:28.

9. Solomon, *True to Our Feelings*, 105.

10. Robert Solomon made this interesting distinction between jealousy and envy. Jealousy is the emotion we feel when something we believe we have a right to is threatened. Envy is the same kind of emotion, except that we know we have no right to the object of the emotion. See Solomon, *True to Our Feelings*, 105. For example, when a musician sees another musician's success, she might feel jealousy or envy. If she has practiced equally and done all the hard work that the successful musician has done, she could feel jealousy because she legitimately has a claim to that kind of success. But if she hasn't done the hard work of preparation, she can feel only envy because she hasn't invested the time and effort and has no right to the claim. Solomon is sometimes associated with the cognitive theory of emotions, which suggests that

we aren't at the mercy of emotions and that with reflection we can evaluate and even alter our emotional state.

11. Chris Tiegreen, *Feeling like God: The Emotional Side of Discipleship—and Why You Can't Fully Follow Jesus without It* (Carol Stream, IL: SaltRiver, 2008), 49.

12. Solomon, *True to Our Feelings*, 111.

CHAPTER 12

1. I lost the source for this interview long ago, but a number of op-eds and articles from the time present a similar perspective. See Mary Brophy Marcus, "Bin Laden's Death a Turning Point for Millennials," *USA Today*, May 4, 2011, http://usatoday30.usatoday.com/yourlife/mind-soul/2011-05-04-bin-laden-youth -millennials_n.htm; Alexandra Petri, "Why We Millennials Celebrated When Osama Died," Opinions, *Washington Post*, May 2, 2011, www.washingtonpost .com/blogs/compost/post/why-we-millennials-celebrated-when-osama-died /2011/03/03/AFx9TMcF_blog.html?utm_term=.a4c6aa70ea86; "Osama bin Laden: The Millennials' Lord Voldemort?," *Week*, May 5, 2011, http://theweek.com/articles/485027/osama-bin-laden-millennials-lord-voldemort.

2. In 2015, the Chapman University Survey of American Fears (Wave 2) cataloged the self-reported fears of our nation. It's a frightening list! See Sheri Ledbetter, "America's Top Fears 2015," Chapman University blog, October 13, 2015, https://blogs.chapman.edu/wilkinson/2015/10/13/americas-top-fears-2015/.

3. A quick count in the NIV of some words I arbitrarily chose: *fear*, *fearful*, *afraid*, *terror*, and *anxious*. There are other words, meaning this is the low end of the possible count.

4. Psalm 23:4.

5. Psalm 27:1.

6. First Peter 5:7 NIV.

7. Psalm 112:1.

8. Psalm 33:18.

9. See John 10:10.

10. "Strong's H3372—*yare*," Blue Letter Bible, accessed May 17, 2017, www.blueletterbible.org/lang/lexicon/Lexicon.cfm?Strongs=H3372&t=KJV.

11. "Strong's H3374—*yir'ah*," Blue Letter Bible, accessed May 17, 2017, www.blueletterbible.org/lang/lexicon/lexicon.cfm?Strongs=H3374.

12. Romans 8:37–39.

13. Robert C. Solomon, *True to Our Feelings: What Our Emotions Are Really Telling Us* (New York: Oxford University Press, 2007), 45.

CHAPTER 13

1. Robert Solomon put it succinctly: "Grief cannot be excluded from the good life even if it is one of the most painful and devastating emotions. If loving and caring are essential to life, then so is grief, which is nothing less than the realization of our extreme vulnerability to loss." Robert C. Solomon, *True to Our Feelings: What Our Emotions Are Really Telling Us* (New York: Oxford University Press, 2007), 72.

2. Byron Kehler is a trauma therapist with more than thirty years of experience working with people who have some of the most painful stories imaginable. Sitting with people in those situations for so long has given him enormous wisdom. I hope he writes his own book someday.

3. Kahlil Gibran, "On Joy and Sorrow," in *The Prophet* (Ware, UK: Wordsworth Editions, 1996), 16.

4. Solomon, *True to Our Feelings*, 74.

5. This passage is quoted in every gospel, as well as in Acts, Romans, and the writings of Peter. It seems notable that a passage highlighting Jesus' emotional struggle and apparent weakness would be that important to the people who originally chronicled His life and ministry. Too often we portray Jesus as a superhero, a man's man, as though He were the most popular kid in high school. But that just makes Him more distant from most of us. This passage tells us that Jesus had many of the same difficulties we do. He wasn't attractive or impressive in person. Some hated Him, and others rejected Him. He experienced suffering. And that's all without factoring in the brutality of His arrest and crucifixion. Jesus' life experience was much closer than we think to the painful lives many of us have had.

6. Isaiah 53:3 ASV.

7. John 11:17–21.

8. Steven Shomler is a former pastor who has worked through enormous personal pain in his own life. You can see him discuss this principle with his son Zac as they talk about the tragic death of his other son, Zayne. Zac Shomler and Steven Shomler, "Crying Is like Going to the Bathroom," *What's Up Shom*, ep. 7, pt. 4, YouTube video, 14:18, posted by Zac Shomler, June 16, 2016, https://youtu.be/VQbZP0qyYn4.

9. Ana Vitlic et al., "Bereavement Reduces Neutrophil Oxidative Burst Only in Older Adults: Role of the HPA Axis and Immunesenescence," *Immunity and*

Ageing 11 (August 2014), www.ncbi.nlm.nih.gov/pmc/articles/PMC4154898/pdf/1742-4933-11-13.pdf.

10. Joseph Bayly, *The View from a Hearse: A Christian View of Death* (Elgin, IL: David C Cook, 1969), 40–41.

11. Romans 12:15.

12. These recommended books, along with many other resources, can be found at www.TheWisdomOfYourHeart.com.

13. According to Robert Solomon, "Many philosophers now argue (as I have) that most emotions are 'rationally assessable' and involve complex motives, goals, intentions, and actions. But this poses a problem for grief, which seems to include a straightforwardly irrational desire—namely, wanting the deceased to come back to life—and therefore produces no intelligible goal or intention, and no action. Grief, unlike most emotions, seemed to entail no actions but rather withdrawal and an inability to do much of anything at all." Solomon, *True to Our Feelings*, 76.

14. This view of grief is an extension of C. S. Lewis' genius argument from desire about the nature of reality. His book *Mere Christianity* lays out this profound argument based on the nature of longing. In nature, creatures are born with desires and needs for certain things they must have, and those things all exist. He wrote the following: "Creatures are not born with desires unless satisfaction for those desires exists. A baby feels hunger: well, there is such a thing as food. A duckling wants to swim: well, there is such a thing as water. Men feel sexual desire: well, there is such a thing as sex. If I find in myself a desire which no experience in this world can satisfy, the most probable explanation is that I was made for another world. If none of my earthly pleasures satisfy it, that does not prove that the universe is a fraud. Probably earthly pleasures were never meant to satisfy it, but only to arouse it, to suggest the real thing." C. S. Lewis, *Mere Christianity* (New York: HarperOne, 2001), 136–37. Lewis expanded on this in *The Weight of Glory*.

15. Psalm 147:3.

16. Revelation 21:4.

CHAPTER 14

1. *Merriam-Webster OnLine*, s.v. "happy," accessed May 17, 2017, www.merriam-webster.com/dictionary/happy.

2. Dr. Carol Ryff proposed that well-being is made up of six dimensions: self-acceptance, environmental mastery, positive relations, purpose in life, personal growth, and autonomy. The higher a person's sense that these factors

are active in his or her life, the more likely that person will be to self-identify as experiencing well-being. While there isn't a direct correlation to happiness, for most people it seems as if the two ideas are synonymous. Carol D. Ryff and Corey Lee M. Keyes, "The Structure of Psychological Well-Being Revisited," *Journal of Personality and Social Psychology* 69, no. 4 (October 1995): 719–27, http://psycnet.apa.org/psycinfo/1996-08070-001.

3. Romans 8:28, which is nearly always quoted out of context. "Work together for the good" refers to the glory that is going to be revealed as God's redemption does its work. Verse 28 culminates an argument that starts with verse 18. Too often Romans 8:28 is quoted to mean that bad things that happen to Christians will always "turn out well" in some way.

4. James Strong, *The New Strong's Complete Dictionary of Bible Words* (Nashville: Thomas Nelson, 1996), 121.

5. In fact, several translations make this very choice, including the Holman Christian Standard Bible (HCSB) and the New Revised Standard Version (NRSV).

6. Matthew 5:3–5 NIV.

7. James 1:2–3.

8. Philippians 4:11–12.

9. Philippians 4:13.

10. See 1 Thessalonians 4:3–8 and 1 Peter 1:13–16 for just two examples.

11. Micah 6:8.

12. First John 1:9.

13. Ephesians 4:32.

14. Galatians 5:22–23.

15. Ephesians 4:13.

16. Eric Hoffer, *The Passionate State of Mind and Other Aphorisms* (New York: Harper, 1955), 151.

17. Psalm 37:1–2.

18. Psalm 37:3.

19. Psalm 37:4.

CHAPTER 15

1. The full quote is rich: "Compassion asks us to go where it hurts, to enter into places of pain, to share in brokenness, fear, confusion, and anguish. Compassion challenges us to cry out with those in misery, to mourn with those who are lonely, to weep with those in tears. Compassion requires us to be weak with the weak, vulnerable with the vulnerable, and powerless with the powerless. Compassion means full immersion in the condition of being human." Henri J. M. Nouwen, Donald P. McNeill, and Douglas A. Morrison, *Compassion: A Reflection on the Christian Life* (New York: Doubleday, 1983), 3–4.

2. First John 4:8.

3. John 3:16.

4. First Corinthians 13:4–8.

5. "Dear friends, let us love one another, because love is from God, and everyone who loves has been born of God and knows God. The one who does not love does not know God, because God is love" (1 John 4:7–8).

6. "No one has ever seen God. If we love one another, God remains in us and His love is perfected in us" (1 John 4:12).

7. See Matthew 5:43–45.

8. James 2:16.

9. It's interesting to note that the person who really noticed this problem we have with *agape* was emotional theorist Robert Solomon, who wasn't a Christian. He wrote, "I mentioned that *agapé* in Christian theology became increasingly idealized, to the point where it became an emotion possible only for God." Robert C. Solomon, *True to Our Feelings: What Our Emotions Are Really Telling Us* (New York: Oxford University Press, 2007), 63.

10. *Online Etymology Dictionary*, s.v. "compassion," accessed May 25, 2015, www.etymonline.com/index.php?term=compassion.

11. Romans 12:15.

12. John 3:16–17.

13. Matthew 1:23.

CHAPTER 16

1. First Kings 19:12 ASV.

2. Luke 8:26–39.

3. Peter Scazzero, *Emotionally Healthy Spirituality: Unleash a Revolution in Your Life in Christ* (Nashville: Thomas Nelson, 2006), 71.

CHAPTER 17

1. Peter Scazzero, *Emotionally Healthy Spirituality: Unleash a Revolution in Your Life in Christ* (Nashville: Thomas Nelson, 2006), 26.

2. Dan B. Allender and Tremper Longman III, *The Cry of the Soul: How Our Emotions Reveal Our Deepest Questions about God* (Colorado Springs, CO: NavPress, 1994), 25.

3. Scazzero, *Emotionally Healthy Spirituality*, 7.

4. Psalm 95:7–8.

5. Ezekiel 36:26.

6. Galatians 5:22–23.

ABOUT THE AUTHOR

Marc Alan Schelske is a husband, dad, speaker, writer, hobbyist theologian, and recovering fundamentalist who drinks tea and rides a motorcycle. He's an avid reader, researcher, and connector of dots.

He is privileged to serve as the teaching elder for Bridge City Community Church, a ragtag faith community in Milwaukie, Oregon. There he focuses on inside-out living and what it looks like to follow Jesus at the intersection of grace and growth. A life-long follower of Jesus, Marc was raised in a pastor's family in the tangled center of a conservative small-church community. In more than two decades of full-time ministry, Marc has had the opportunity to experience the good and bad of Christian leadership and community. He's also walked through the full range of pastoral-care situations, learning the questions people really ask and the problems they really face.

As a writer and speaker, Marc brings creativity, passion, and solid Bible study with theological depth, as well as a vulnerable and authentic voice that connects with people worn out by the church machine. In addition to this book, Marc is the author of *Discovering*

Your Authentic Core Values: A Step-by-Step Guide, as well as several online discipleship and personal-growth courses, including "Not Just One More Thing: Spiritual Growth for Busy People" and "How to Read the Bible to Hear God and Grow, without Having to Be a Legalist, a Theology Professor, or a Crackpot," that can be found at www.TheApprenticeshipLab.com. Marc has a bachelor of arts degree in theology from Walla Walla University.

More important than any of this, however, Marc has walked the difficult path of emotional recovery. Growing up in a conservative, traditional church community, he internalized many messages about avoiding, ignoring, or repressing emotions. Trauma early in life and his own perfectionism wired him for a driven life of accomplishment and performance.

In 2006, with the birth of his first child, his life began to splinter and fall apart, leaving Marc in a deep depression. His emotionally disconnected life very nearly cost him everything that mattered to him—his marriage, his family, his ministry. Step by step, with the care of wise mentors, a grace-filled community, miles of painful personal exploration, and the guidance of a caring therapist, Marc has walked through his own darkness, experiencing the ongoing fruit of a spiritual life that includes emotional growth.

Marc would love to hear from you. You can find him and his writing at www.MarcAlanSchelske.com and get connected on Twitter (@Schelske) and Facebook (www.Facebook.com/MarcAlanSchelske).

At David C Cook, we equip the local church around
the corner and around the globe to make disciples.
Come see how we are working together—go to
www.davidccook.com. Thank you!

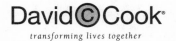

transforming lives together